Get into nursing and midwifery

Get into nursing and midwifery

A guide to application and career success

Sarah Snow
University of Worcester

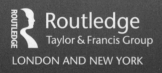
Routledge
Taylor & Francis Group

LONDON AND NEW YORK

First published 2012 by Pearson Education Limited

Published 2013 by Routledge
2 Park Square, Milton Park, Abingdon, Oxon OX14 4RN
711 Third Avenue, New York, NY 10017, USA

Routledge is an imprint of the Taylor & Francis Group, an informa business

ISBN 13: 978-0-273-74609-6 (pbk)

British Library Cataloguing-in-Publication Data
A catalogue record for this book is available from the British Library

Library of Congress Cataloguing-in-Publication Data
Snow, Sarah, 1966-
  Get into nursing and midwifery : a guide to application and career success / Sarah Snow.
      p. ; cm.
  Includes bibliographical references and index.
  ISBN 978-0-273-74609-6 (pbk.)
  I. Title.
  [DNLM: 1. Career Choice. 2. Nursing. 3. Midwifery. WY 16.1]

618.2--dc23

                                          2011043052
Typeset in 9/13 Interstate by 73

For Bella and Maddy
My Star Girls

2014002468

Contents

Preface

This book is aimed at prospective students who wish to enter the nursing or midwifery professions. It has been written in response to the significant increase in applications to these courses and is meant to be especially helpful to those wishing to compete for a place on oversubscribed programmes such as midwifery and child health nursing. A guide such as this is therefore timely and should serve as an invaluable and friendly companion through the varied challenges that lie ahead for those wishing to enter the professions.

Nursing and midwifery are among the top five most popular course choices according to UCAS and their appeal has endured over time. The reasons for this appeal are explored in this book, although they must also be viewed within a broader demographic context. The UK recession and generalised slump in the world economy has forced many people to re-evaluate where they are going in life and how best to seek long-term job satisfaction. Although nursing and midwifery can no longer afford the same level of job security they once did, the professions still maintain a specific appeal because of the challenging yet rewarding nature of caring for others, together with the wide ranging career opportunities that can arise for nurses and midwives at the point of registration.

A recent Higher Education Policy Institute report (Bekhradnia and Bailey, 2008) suggests that the number of 18-year-olds in the population is likely to have peaked during 2010, meaning that the demand for university places will remain high for at least the immediate future. This population growth has resulted in a threefold increase in applications to some universities, the result being intense competition for highly popular ones such as midwifery. Although many parents would aspire for their children to attend university, a large number will be disappointed this year and very likely over the next few, as the level of competition remains high and the number of university places available either fall or remain the same. This situation is likely to be exacerbated by the sharp increase in university tuition fees for non-professional courses.

How will this book help alleviate some of this angst? Hopefully in several constructive and helpful ways. It is written in the sequence that applicants follow during their journey into a healthcare profession and therefore addresses the crucial issues associated with application, shortlisting and selection. The various parts of the book are supported by contributions from authors who have interest and expertise in issues that affect undergraduate students generally, and healthcare profession students specifically. These contributions are weaved through text that is intended to be supportive, encouraging and above all else, realistic. It is not an academic textbook, rather one that is based on the author's professional experience, knowledge and skills that have been amassed over numerous years in clinical practice and education. The writing style is deliberately informal and friendly to invite the reader in and encourage them to stay. Each section contains top tips and frequently, specific tools that will help the reader in their journey towards their place on a professional course.

Although the focus of this book is nursing and midwifery, much of the advice offered could apply to other healthcare professions, for example paramedics or social care, as some of the guidance and information can easily be applied to those settings. Although this book is not a guarantee of a place on a highly desired healthcare course, it will serve as a faithful, reliable companion through the many challenges that lie ahead on the road to professional registration.

List of contributors

Sarah Holling, BSc (Hons), MA, Chartered MCIPD

Sarah Holling is a second year adult nursing student at the University of Surrey. She has over 15 years' HR experience in the UK and abroad, including graduate recruitment, selection centre design, psychometric testing and advising young people on employment and training. Sarah has also managed university admissions for postgraduate mental health programmes.

Jo Rouse, RGN, RSCN, MSc, FHEA, RNT

Jo Rouse is a senior lecturer and programme lead for pre-registration nursing at the University of Worcester. Her professional expertise is in teaching child protection and reflective practice in nursing. Jo has extensive experience as an admissions/induction tutor for pre-registration nursing students.

Kim Russell, MA, PG Cert (HE), BSc (Hons), RM, RGN

Kim Russell is a senior lecturer and senior teaching Fellow at the University of Worcester. She has many years of experience, both as a community midwife and educator where her aim is to prepare students for professional practice and develop their capacity to lead and enlarge the midwifery profession. Kim's doctoral research centres on improving hospital midwives' confidence in water birth practice.

Martin Spurin, NEBSM, HND, BSc, MEd

Martin Spurin is a lecturer at University College Birmingham. Although he has led a range of programmes in many disciplines, he currently manages the part-time foundation degree and degree programme in Community Family Support. His first degree was in hospitality and his Masters was in Education. Martin is currently doing doctoral research which focuses on mature students returning to part time education.

Key facts

- Successful completion of an approved programme of nurse or mid-wife education leads to the dual awards of a degree/diploma and professional registration with the Nursing and Midwifery Council (NMC).

- Student nurses and midwives must satisfy the clinical and theoretical requirements of their educational programmes, set by the NMC and known as the Standards for Pre-Registration Nursing/Midwifery Education (NMC, 2009; 2010).

- At the point of registration, nurses and midwives are accountable for their practice and adhere to NMC standards and guidelines. All registered practitioners (and students) abide by the NMC Code (NMC, 2008). This means that you are obliged to:

  - Make the care of people your first concern, treating them as individuals and respecting their dignity;
  - Work with others to protect and promote the health and well being of those in your care, their families and carers, and the wider community;
  - Provide a high standard of practice and care at all times;
  - Be open and honest, act with integrity and uphold the reputation of your profession.

- Students on undergraduate programmes in England are entitled to apply for an income-assessed bursary via the NHS Business Services Authority (http://www.nhsbsa.nhs.uk/Students/816.aspx), and a student loan. For students living elsewhere in the UK, the arrangements are broadly comparable. From September 2012, nursing and midwifery students will also receive a £1000 grant.

- All applications to nursing and midwifery programmes are made via UCAS each year during a defined application cycle (http://www.ucas.com/).

- As at April 2011, salaries for newly qualified nurses and midwives start at £21,176 (band 5). High cost areas, such as London, will add on a salary supplement, for example up to 20 per cent.

Acknowledgements

I am extremely grateful to all my professional colleagues who have made such helpful and informative contributions to this book. That this was done as a favour to me during intensely busy times at work and within the context of major political change in the NHS and higher education makes me especially grateful and appreciative – thank you very much.

I am also indebted to all the midwifery and nursing students who enthusiastically shared their own stories, read extracts and offered suggestions, thus enabling me to weave those insights into the book and ensure that my advice and suggestions to the reader are 'real'.

Thanks also to David Harrison and Helen Leech at Pearson, the former who recognised the potential for a book of this kind from an early stage, and the latter who steered me along the right path and was consistent in her prompt feedback and encouraging support. As a newcomer to the book writing game, I appreciated this stewardship as it was done with skill and sensitivity and above all else, enabled me freedom during the development and writing of the book.

Chapter 1

An introduction to the professions

Learning outcomes

By the end of Chapter 1, you should be able to:

- ✔ understand the key differences between nursing and midwifery
- ✔ recognise the essential skills and attributes required of a nurse or midwife and why they are important
- ✔ begin to relate those skills and attributes to your own
- ✔ appreciate the impact a nurse or midwife has on the well-being and experiences of healthcare consumers
- ✔ confidently identify your chosen professional route and continue relevant research using the resources provided

Introduction

This opening chapter explores the nature of the nursing and midwifery professions, what it means to be a nurse or midwife, and what sort of essential skills and attributes are required. Rather than do this as a lengthy, descriptive account that can tend to be rather dry, I have instead enlisted the help of colleagues who between them have created rich and varied accounts of their professional lives and the nature of the patients/clients they serve. These should serve to illuminate the professions and can be placed in further context later on in the chapter by reading the perspectives of students themselves.

Why be a nurse or midwife?

Chapter 1 is important in helping towards the development of knowledge and understanding of your chosen profession. As you will discover in Chapter 3, being able to articulate a clear and objective motivation for application to a nursing or midwifery degree programme is key to being successful at the shortlisting stage. This section will therefore focus on the essential characteristics of nurses and midwives, illuminated by reflections on practice from clinicians, their typical 'life in a day' diaries, and by the perspectives of nursing students. Firstly, it is important to place this within a broad historical context as both people and policies continue to have a significant influence on healthcare, and therefore practitioners, in contemporary Britain.

There are a number of excellent texts available that outline the historical development of the professions – details of these are provided in the next section. As part of the research into your chosen profession and certainly before you apply for a place on a highly competitive course, you would be wise to look at some of these first. Not only will this background reading be interesting and relevant to your application, it is an important step in the decision-making process. Although a detailed history of the professions is outside the remit of this book (and has been done very well by many others), it may be of use to you to complete a historical timeline of important events. Your background reading, guided by the references provided, will help illuminate these events and enrich your understanding of the profession you have chosen to apply for.

Historical timeline

The key resources provided in Box 1.1 will help you understand the events on the timeline and to complete the blank sections in Activity 1.1. Completing this activity will provide valuable information for future reference, as well as being a way of developing your information searching skills. Spaces have been left at the end of the table for you to add anything else that you consider relevant during completion of the timeline. As a midwife teacher, I know that information gathering is an essential skill for undergraduate midwifery and nursing students to acquire early on in their studies – so why not start now.

Box 1.1 Timeline resources

Lowis G, van Tejilingen E, McCaffery P, Porter M (eds) (2004) *Midwifery and the Medicalisation of Childbirth: Comparative Perspectives.* Nova Science Publishers Inc.

http://www.bbc.co.uk/radio4/womanshour/02/2009_24_tue.shtml
BBC Radio Woman's Hour broadcast about the history of district nursing.

http://www.nmc-uk.org/About-us/The-history-of-nursing-and-midwifery-regulation/
NMC page looking at the history of nursing and midwifery regulation.

http://www.nursing.manchester.ac.uk/ukchnm/
UK Centre for the History of Nursing and Midwifery.

ACTIVITY 1.1

Historical timeline

Research the events listed and then make notes in the spaces available.

Date	Event	Notes
1858	Registration of the medical profession began	
1881	Mary Seacole died	
1902	Midwives Registration Act	
1910	Florence Nightingale died	
1919	Nurses Registration Act	
1948	NHS came into effect	
1970	The Peel Report	
1972	The Briggs Report	
1979	Nurses, Midwives and Health Visitors Act	
1983	UKCC established	
1985	Introduction of Project 2000 Nurse Education	
1989	The Children's Act	
1993	'Changing Childbirth' report published	
2000	The NHS Plan published	
2002	NMC replaced the UKCC	
2010	Coalition Government proposes NHS reform	

🕐 What is it like being a nurse or midwife?

In order to answer this question, I have drawn together a number of personal reflections and diary extracts from colleagues who have amassed a vast number of years' experience between them as healthcare practitioners. These will offer the reader a 'bird's-eye' view of what makes a nurse or midwife tick.

Names of clients/patients are pseudonyms in order to protect confidentiality.

Sarah Snow, Midwife

My career in healthcare began by accident in 1984. As a naïve 18-year-old, I had no real idea of what I wished to do with my life – nursing seemed as good a job as any, although I remember that my Dad really wanted me to work in a bank. In those days, dual registration was considered to be an excellent career move and I therefore embarked on a midwifery pathway after some experience as a Staff nurse. I have little memory of my training, other than being told off on a regular basis – in those days, nursing and midwifery was strictly hierarchical and regimental. I frequently breached the 'rules' by making friends with the night sisters, or having my hair longer than the top of my uniform collar. It's really only the experiences I subsequently enjoyed as a qualified midwife that began to shape my philosophy about the care of women during childbirth and the importance of looking after student midwives.

In 1994, I was working on the delivery suite of a maternity unit that handled around 1,500 births per year. I had been qualified as a midwife for four years and was just starting to have the confidence to assert myself more as the midwife I wanted to be. I believed, and still do, that women should do what feels right for them during the births of their babies, but was also acutely aware that women's wishes were frequently ignored or sidetracked within the maternity services. I was happy working within this maternity unit and felt supported and valued in my practice most

Reflection 1.1

of the time. It was also a significant time in my personal life – I got married and met my closest friend through working at this unit. In addition, two of my current teaching colleagues who I respect greatly were also midwives within the unit at this time.

During one particular shift, I looked after Jill, who was in labour having her second baby. I hadn't met Jill before – this was usual – and therefore had limited time to foster an effective relationship with her. As we got to know each other a little, Jill told me that her first experience had been mostly negative – she felt little choice had been offered, and her birth plan not respected. We talked about Jill's wishes for the delivery of this baby and she asked me, very tentatively, if she could give birth standing up. I had not helped women in this position before, and knew that many of my colleagues were sceptical about any position other than being on a delivery bed, but I was very happy to support Jill in her wish – it really didn't seem to be a big deal for me.

A few hours later, Jill delivered her baby girl standing up with me crouching at her feet ready to catch the baby. The baby was born very quickly and easily because of the upright position – I learnt for the next time to encourage women to lean forwards slightly to slow down the birth a little – and Jill was absolutely delighted and full of praise for me. I remember thinking 'why is she so grateful?' because all I had done was support Jill in her decision-making. Of course, as I got older and somewhat wiser, I realised that my small contribution to this woman's birth was hugely significant in terms of her choice and control. This significance was reinforced during the births of my own children, where the need to emerge emotionally intact from the experience was hugely important to me.

Later, I received a card from Jill that thanked me for making her birth 'so unfrightening'. There was also a gift – a beautiful Art Deco mug that sits on my shelves still, 16 years later. Seeing it there serves as a beacon of light in my ongoing practice as a midwifery educator. It takes courage to support women's choices within hostile birth environments, especially with the knowledge that the application of that courage can have life-long consequences.

Pete Stenson, Nurse Specialist, Sexual Health

It is not uncommon for patients to ask 'what made you choose this job?' Perhaps the patient would like to hear that it was a calling and that the nurse 'just wanted to help sick people' when in fact the reason may be geographical: 'I only live around the corner'; financial: 'this job pays more'; or social: 'the hours fit in with childcare'. Sometimes, patients state 'Oh I couldn't do your job'. I've never been quite sure if this is supposed to make nurses feel better about their career choice.

Like many nurses, I was directly influenced in my choice by my experience as a student nurse. In the late 1960s, it was felt by nurse tutors that it was inappropriate for male students to have placements on the gynaecological wards, so I was sent along to what was then called the 'VD Clinic'. The clinic was to be found in the basement next to the boiler house and the entrance was separate from the main outpatient entrance. The small door in the wall had a sign above it that proclaimed 'Chest Clinic'. I thought the rather dingy setting did not bode well for a six-week placement. Nothing could have been further from the truth. The inside of the clinic was clean and bright and the staff happy and smiling. I reported to Mr Jack Edwards, the nurse/technician who was in charge of the clinic. Not only was he very welcoming, he immediately gave me a tour of the clinic and introduced me to the other staff, including the consultant who also welcomed me to the clinic. In my previous ward experience, I don't think that a consultant had ever spoken directly to me, so this was a novel experience. The training programme was explained to me – it included some real hands-on stuff like microscopy, issuing medicines, requesting microbiology tests and taking blood; the latter were tasks at that time only undertaken by doctors. Being the only student, I was given individual tuition and I responded by even reading about sexually transmitted diseases in my own time!

I followed Jack Edwards around for the first few weeks and was amazed by his in-depth knowledge – on occasion, even the consultant sought his opinion. The range of duties he was able to carry out was extensive and he took decisions about the diagnosis and what treatment the patient was to receive. But above all I was struck by his kindness to the patients, many of whom were devastated when told that they had a sexually acquired infection. At that time, the stigma and risks surrounding these diseases were very real.

My six happy weeks in the clinic soon came to an end. Before I left, Jack took me to one side to explain all the benefits that working in the clinic would have once I had completed my training – his memorable comment was that 'as long as people had sex I would always have a job'. He painted a rosy picture of life in what he called the 'Cinderella service'. I took him at his word; I started work in sexual health in the early 1970s and have continued in the same job for 38 years. Everything Jack had predicted turned out to be true; sexual health nurses have a good deal of autonomy and nurse led services now make up the majority of clinic appointments.

It is quite trendy to work in sexual health now and I have enjoyed introducing numerous students to the delights of sexual health nursing. I had the honour of working with Jack for five years until he retired aged 81. Many years later, when we moved to new premises I had the pleasure of naming the new clinic after him.

Ali Spencer, Critical Care Outreach Sister

Life-in-a-day 1.1

I am part of a Critical Care Outreach Team in a District General Hospital. The team was set up 11 years ago as a government initiative to provide support and education to general ward nurses looking after deteriorating patients on general wards. It is made up of senior nurses who have all had several years of Critical Care experience and who are also experienced in teaching and supporting other nurses.

It is a fantastic job as it allows me to care for really sick patients and to teach other nurses, which are both passions of mine!

To give you some insight into my role I thought I would share a few hours of a typical day with you and hopefully you'll agree that it is interesting and exciting.

It is Saturday morning and I arrive for work at 8.40 am to find my partner in crime for the day waiting for me in the office. He has already taken handover from the Night Nurse Practitioner who has asked him to see one patient that she had been called to overnight. He has also been to the Critical Care Unit to find that two patients were discharged to general wards overnight. Our hours of service are 8.00 am to 5.00 pm every day and we work closely with the Night Nurse Practitioners so that nurses can be supported caring for sick patients 24 hours a day. We see all patients who are discharged from the Critical Care Unit and also take referrals from ward nurses, specialist nurses and doctors. Once we have identified and allocated the patients to be seen, we set off to assess them. We carry one pager each that allows doctors and nurses to contact us to refer sick patients, and also the Medical Emergency pager as we form part of that team also.

My first patient is a gentleman who was discharged from the Critical Care Unit yesterday afternoon to a general surgical ward. He is 72 years old and had undergone bowel surgery for a tumour. He required critical care support because he had a history of cardiac disease and stroke but he had an uneventful recovery and now requires follow up from Outreach.

I arrived on the ward and introduced myself to him and to the nurse looking after him, before carrying out a comprehensive assessment including observations and test results. I found him to be recovering well and only needed to reduce his oxygen and advise on frequency of observations before reassuring him of his good progress. He was quite straightforward as he had only been a patient on the unit for 24 hours. I discharged him to the care of the ward staff but reassured them that they could contact me about him if they became concerned about his condition.

Some patients are on the Critical Care Unit for days, even weeks, and as a result may suffer psychological problems such as anxiety, sleeplessness, hallucinations, memory loss and confusion. It is vital that these patients are supported by nurses who understand the problems they are experiencing and are able to reassure and encourage them in their recovery. The Outreach team can be very important in these instances as we have lots of experience of looking after patients with these problems. I have looked after many patients who have vivid memories of their stay in Critical Care – often, these memories take the form of frightening dreams or hallucinations. I recall one gentleman who had experienced disturbing hallucinations and felt frightened and unsure of all staff. The ward staff found it very difficult to reassure him and they all needed a lot of support and encouragement. I was able to explain his hallucinations to the nurses and then reassure the patient that although very vivid to him, they were not real. I was also able to take him back to the Unit once he was medically stable to show him around and it helped him to remember some of the things that had really happened.

While on the ward a Nursing Auxiliary asked if I could teach him how to record a manual blood pressure as he had not carried out this task for a while. I explained the process to him, demonstrated the technique and then observed as he practised. He was most grateful and set off to practise! Next I had to return to the office in order to synchronise the hand-held device that we use to record patient information and assessment onto the database on the computer. This then allows for a printout to be made of the assessment and suggestions that can then be filed in the patient's notes as a reminder to all staff caring for the patient. I was on my way to file the sheet when the Medical Emergency bleep went off and I had to speed along to a ward where an elderly gentleman had suffered a cardiac arrest. I helped the anaesthetist to establish a safe airway and performed cardiopulmonary resuscitation (CPR). Unfortunately the gentleman didn't recover and after 30 minutes it was agreed that the resuscitation should stop and the gentleman died shortly afterwards.

The next patient was a 19-year-old boy with motor neurone disease who had been admitted to the general respiratory ward with a chest infection. He was normally cared for at home by his mother who took care of all his needs and managed him in a wheelchair. He was able to talk but could not manage any of his own care. He had already experienced one previous admission to Critical Care where he needed help to breathe with a ventilator, so it was important that his condition was monitored closely. On arrival, his mother was in attendance and explained that she was very anxious and concerned about him and felt that he was getting worse. It can be very distressing for people who are caring for their relatives at home in a familiar environment when they have to be admitted to hospital. All of a sudden their routine and environment is different and they are expected to fit into a completely different one. She described feeling out of control and fearful of what would happen if her son continued to deteriorate. I was able to reassure her that we would take very good care of him and that I would assess him and monitor for signs of deterioration. I could then liaise with the doctors in his team on the ward and also the Critical Care Anaesthetists in case he needed to be admitted for more intensive care.

I carried out a full clinical assessment, at all times explaining my actions and reassuring the young man that he was in safe hands. Unfortunately he did show signs of clinical deterioration and I had to contact a senior doctor in his team. Tests indicated that he was not breathing adequately and consequently, I called the Anaesthetist to assess him for admission to the Critical Care Unit.

During this process, I was able to reassure the patient and his mother as the situation changed, and also to support and facilitate the ward nurse looking after him. I liaised with both the doctors in charge of his care and also the Critical Care Anaesthetist in an attempt to plan and manage the best care for the patient. This is a really good example of the benefit of having a Critical Care Outreach team, as it is extremely important that there is someone who can understand the situation from all angles and then communicate with all disciplines of staff involved.

It was agreed that the young man would be best managed in the Critical Care Unit and so I prepared him for transfer using the appropriate equipment and safely transferred him to the Unit with his mother close behind. I helped to settle him into the Unit and gave handover to the nurse who was to look after him there before showing his mother to the waiting room.

Once he was safely settled in I set off to lunch – presuming that the pager didn't go off!!

Jo Jones, Education and Development Facilitator

07.30: Arrive in the office. Spend some time replying to emails relating to planned teaching sessions, student and preceptee[1] support and allocations of students within practice areas, as well as arranging various meetings that have been requested overnight – it is surprising how many people email overnight!

08.30: Set up the rooms for teaching today. We have a Preceptorship group in this morning. It is the launch of our new programme – with 25 Newly Qualified Practitioners taking up employment, this promises to be a full year ahead. I enjoy these first few days the most as they provide valuable time to get to know each other, especially as we will work so closely together over the forthcoming year or so (as well as time to catch up with students who we already know who left here just a couple of months ago in a very different role!).

09.00: We welcome our new group of preceptees to our programme with some fun icebreaker games and choccies – a great way to start any day!!

11.00: Break for coffee. Quick dash back to the office as I am keen to check if there are any further attendances confirmed at this afternoon's taught session relating to Documentation and Record Keeping. It is the first of ten planned sessions that, together, form a newly developed programme for our midwifery students. I developed the programme alongside two midwifery lecturers, and this is therefore an exciting time for all three of us. The entire programme content has been organised in response to student and preceptee needs and therefore only time will measure our success here. There were 12 attendances confirmed this morning and another three now – really pleased so far.

11.30: Coffee break over and we recommence the Preceptorship launch. The next period is planned time to consider the forthcoming Preceptorship period for the Newly Qualified Practitioners.

This time provides us all with the opportunity to sit and discuss hopes, fears and expectations of their first year as qualified, autonomous practitioners. It is good to see that it is no surprise to any of the group that the forthcoming year is going to be another steep learning curve, but all seem to be excited and enthusiastic about the next stage of their professional journeys!

13.00: Lunchtime sees the end of today's teaching for me. Time now to finish catching up in the office and then set up for this afternoon's session. I have received a couple of requests regarding Mentorship Preparation courses and a request to return a call to a student in further education who wishes to embark on a career in midwifery. I return her call and we discuss the options available to her as well as ways to move forward towards her chosen career. Hopefully, her application will be successful and we will meet in the near future.

13.30: Attendance at the Documentation and Record Keeping session is fantastic. By attending this programme, midwifery students from all cohorts have an opportunity to learn and develop from each other, supported by the guidance and expertise of a very experienced Supervisor of Midwives[2] with a particular interest in the subject and who has kindly given her time to deliver the session.

15.00: The first session of the new programme has finished and we have received really positive evaluations. Some students presented interesting case studies and experiences for discussion. This helped to ensure that the session was informal, interactive and valuable. Following the close of the session, there was an opportunity to catch up with some students, all of whom tell me that they are enjoying their hospital and community placements. One midwifery student has asked for some support and advice with regards to the achievement of her practice placement requirements throughout the remainder of the semester. I suggest we head over to the placement area to discuss this in more detail with her mentor as well. By doing this, we can ensure that what she plans is realistic and achievable within the available timeframe.

15.30: We arrive on Delivery Suite and take time to discuss the many ways in which she could extend her learning opportunities. Attending a variety of clinics or visiting other practice areas is always a useful way to optimise learning – new skills can be acquired and knowledge deepened. The maternity ward co-ordinators and I have just completed an audit of the practice areas, so we use this as a guide to the learning opportunities that are available to the midwifery students while on placements in these areas.

16.45: Back to the office now to review plans for tomorrow before heading off for the day. Tomorrow looks to be another busy day as we have a Mentor and Preceptorship Update, alongside making visits to practice placements to support both students and mentors within their clinical areas. I enjoy spending time in the clinical areas meeting both students and qualified staff while they are working in practice. The enthusiasm and eagerness of others to learn and teach becomes most evident here and this is great to see.

Notes

1. A preceptee is a newly qualified nurse, midwife or allied health professional, who undergoes a period of preceptorship in order to facilitate the transition from student to autonomous practitioner. See Department of Health (2010) *Preceptorship Framework for Nurses, Midwives and Allied Health Professionals*, Department of Health, London for more information.

2. A Supervisor of Midwives is an experienced midwife who, following completion of additional training, supports the practice of a nominated group of midwives in order to maintain professional standards and safeguard the public. See **www.nmc-org.uk** for more information.

Philip Jones, Mental Health Nurse

The wonderful thing about working with people is that you can never entirely predict what might happen next. As a mental health nurse I think this is perhaps even truer. I am a team leader in an assertive outreach team, a specialist mental health team working with patients who may need more intensive support, or might be difficult to work with for any number of reasons including previous bad experiences, chaotic lifestyles or lack of permanent housing.

Each day begins with a handover at the office to find out what has gone on during the previous day (or over the weekend). We recount key aspects of our visits to patients focusing on important issues such as whether medication was delivered, if a patient is well or if they may be becoming unwell and what follow up might be required.

There are a variety of other activities that take place and are discussed during some morning meetings:

- Every patient in our care has a care plan with formal reviews every six months to make sure we are doing the right things and to help us identify areas that might no longer be required or need to be done differently. The care we provide to each patient depends on what key needs are identified within the context of the care plan meeting. It is a constant, ongoing process and tailored to the needs of the individual.

- Each patient in mental health services has a care co-ordinator whose job is to plan and make sure the right care is delivered. Sometimes a care co-ordinator might decide that they cannot provide the appropriate care to a patient and so may refer them to us. We would then invite that care co-ordinator over for a meeting with the team as part of our assessment to see if it might be appropriate for us to take over care.

- About once a month we also have a business meeting. This is an opportunity for staff to find out information about what is going on in the wider service, ask questions of managers about practical

Life-in-a-day 1.3

things or for the manager to discuss important issues with the team. This is a positive opportunity to discuss anything from trivial matters about office supply problems to very important issues related to changes expected in the service as a result of the recent economic situation.

- During the meeting every Monday we discuss every patient on our caseload, discuss what happened last week, discuss what needs to be done during the coming week and arrange who will do it.

Once the meeting is finished staff will usually spend some time checking their emails, picking up phone messages and dealing with anything urgent first. On a Monday, we can often be in the office for most of the morning. Much of the meeting is often focused on reflecting on what we have been doing and assessing whether other things are needed.

If we have patients who are becoming unwell, we may need to start to visit more often to try to make sure the patient is taking their medication. If we are very concerned or have already tried to do this, we may need to arrange for our team doctor to go out with another doctor and an approved mental health professional (traditionally a social worker but now sometimes a nurse) to do a Mental Health Act assessment to assess whether the patient might need to be admitted to hospital. After we leave the office, staff will go to see the patients they've agreed to see during the planning meeting. During each visit the member of staff will be assessing the patient's mental health to make sure they are staying well, but the way this is done may vary. Sometimes visits can be very short – just saying a quick hello, perhaps giving the patient their medication for the week. On other occasions we may be spending several hours or even whole days with patients for special reasons. There are a number of visits that we might do during an average day and it depends on the needs and willingness of the patient, for example:

- A social visit might just be a matter of calling around and having a cup of tea with a patient to spend some time chatting with them and maybe also their carer/relatives. During this kind of visit the staff member will make an assessment of the patient's mental health, explore whether there are any specific needs and sometimes as a result of doing this, support the patient in dealing with a matter such as a benefits query. On other occasions the purpose of a social visit may be more specific. We have many patients who are very isolated and lonely for example, who would benefit from activities such as attending a day centre or going for a walk. We might accompany them during such activities in order to spend some time with them. On other occasions we may be trying to enable a patient to do some very ordinary things. Perhaps a patient wants to do some shopping but is very anxious. Spending too much time inside is not good for anyone and so encouraging people to come with us for short walks, to visit the local shop or even go to play snooker, watch football or go to concerts, is all part of our role to enable people to do the ordinary things which they may not feel able to do on their own.

- We have a group of patients who can be very chaotic and disorganised and if a patient has an appointment with a GP or Citizens Advice Bureau for example, we will often offer to attend with them. However, we must always be aware of the patient's rights to privacy and so the level of support will depend on what they want from us and what they will accept. The aim over time is always that the patient will become more independent and therefore need us less.

- We may also visit a patient to offer some specific support, for example helping to complete a housing benefit form, or supporting a patient to do some housework. Many of our patients find it difficult to keep a positive routine in regards to keeping their home environment appropriately tidy, and this can become a further stress for them. As before, the aim is to promote independent living.

- One aspect of our role is offering specific input regarding a patient's mental health. Although most staff lack first-hand experience of mental illness, our experience of working with people means that we often have a plethora of ideas about what we have seen work in the past. Some people find listening to music soothing, whereas others may believe that the radio/CD is speaking to them or about them during times of illness. There is a basic level of advice provided about avoiding large quantities of alcohol and the dangers of illicit substance misuse that are often a contributory factor in the patients that we see. At a more complex level, there is family therapy to assist in helping families to understand their patterns of communication and perhaps learn how to adapt these patterns to avoid some relational difficulties. There are also a variety of psychological therapies available, such as CBT (cognitive behavioural therapy), and work that can be done to help patients understand when they are becoming unwell.

Other than the fact that we finish work at sometime around 5.00 pm each day, every day is different. It is not unusual to travel from a Mental Health Act assessment to play a game of snooker with a patient to finish the day, or to offer some practical advice/support to a carer, or simply to listen to them. It is this variety of work that I have become accustomed to and that means I'm rarely bored!

What skills and attributes do I need to be a nurse or midwife?

This question will be revisited throughout the book, as it is crucial to your understanding of the profession that you are seeking to join and therefore the overall strength of your application and performance at selection. So far, the reflective accounts and life-in-a-day diaries from various healthcare professionals should have given you a very good idea of the key attributes and skills required of a nurse or midwife practitioner in twenty-first-century Britain. Can you think about some of these skills and attributes now and write them down in Activity 1.2?

ACTIVITY 1.2

The key skills and attributes of a nurse and midwife

From your reading so far, list the key skills and attributes of a nurse and midwife:

You can add to this list as your reading expands, and perhaps after speaking to staff at university open days. This task will also help you when it comes to writing the all-important personal statement when you're ready to apply.

As part of the research towards writing this book, the opinions of a group of first-year student nurses were sought. They were asked: 'What are the most important skills/attributes of a nurse?' Their responses are listed in Box 1.2, in descending order of frequency. Do any of them match the ones listed by you in Activity 1.2?

Box 1.2 The most important skills/ attributes of a nurse

1. Communication
2. Compassion
3. Empathy
4. Patience
5. Caring

6. Knowledgeable
7. Sense of humour
8. Open-minded
9. Tough
10. Approachable

CHAPTER 1 ● AN INTRODUCTION TO THE PROFESSIONS

Now that we have begun to identify the skills, knowledge and attributes required of a nurse or midwife practitioner, let's consider some of the specific developments within the professions in order to think more about what it is you want to do and why.

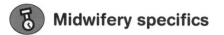 Midwifery specifics

The midwife has been in existence for ever, although she may not necessarily have been known by that name for all of the time. There are references to midwives practising in the Old Testament, ancient Egypt and Rome. Throughout popular culture, art and literature there are representations of midwives, some more flattering than others. Her skills have been praised and celebrated around the world; a guardian and protector of normal birth. However, those skills have also been feared within repressive societies and she has subsequently been the target of persecution. Many of the countless numbers of women burnt at the stake during the purges of the Middle Ages were midwives and/or traditional healers. Their knowledge of the therapeutic properties of certain plants, for example, made them vulnerable to charges of witchcraft. Barbara Ehrenreich and Deirdre English have written excellent accounts of these important historical events and a link to one of them has been provided for you in the Further Reading section at the end of the chapter.

The history and professional regulation of midwifery is quite distinct from that of nursing, and consequently followed a very different professional path. From the work of Donnison (1988), we know the following: Traditionally, women have always cared for other women during childbirth. Often untrained women (and therefore perceived as being unskilled), who were perhaps senior members of the local community, were called upon to help bring new life into the world as well as aid those departing it. For these services, payment was usually 'in kind' or provided free to the poorest families. Childbirth was a hazardous event for women and indeed still is for women who live in the poorer parts of the world, and the presence of a familiar midwife to support and monitor birth, rather than seek to control or interrupt it, significantly reduced this hazard. Poorer women who couldn't afford the services

of doctors or hospitals, instead relying on the local 'handywoman' or
a female relative, had better outcomes than wealthier women, even
though they were often malnourished and exhausted from frequent
childbirth. Ironically, this was probably the only time in a woman's life
when she was better off being poor.

Childbirth shifted dramatically during the latter part of the twentieth
century from home or small maternity 'homes', to hospital, a controver-
sial move that has had huge consequences for birth outcomes and wom-
en's experiences (Donnison, 1988). With the rise in hospital birth came
the consequential rise in the medicalisation of birth and the adoption of
practices that were perceived to be of benefit: the use of drugs to induce
labour and control pain; routine enemas and pubic hair shaving; electronic monitoring of the fetal heart during labour; routine episiotomy;
regulated infant feeding. Many of these practices have since been aban-
doned after evidence demonstrated them to be of no clinical benefit.
However, one consequence of medicalised birth, a dramatic increase in
caesarean section, continues to cause controversy within the professions, as well as creating confusion and anxiety for consumers. Around
24 per cent of babies born today in the UK will be delivered by caesarean section (Bragg et al, 2010) and there is persistent debate about the
impact of this intervention on maternal and neonatal outcomes.

Midwives work in a variety of settings, essentially based around either
the hospital or community. Some midwives have successfully managed to link the two by working in small teams and providing antenatal,
labour and postnatal care to a defined caseload of women. Others work
within maternity units in hospitals, providing the range of midwifery
care but not necessarily to the same women. Many more choose to
work as community midwives where they are able to foster excellent
relationships with women during the antenatal and postnatal periods, and when women choose to give birth at home. The majority of
midwives in the UK operate within the NHS, although there are some
private maternity hospitals. There are also a number of midwives who
practise independently, either alone or in small teams.

As well as enjoying the broad scope of clinical practice, caring for women
throughout the childbirth continuum, midwives also have a broad range
of career opportunities. These include roles in education, research and

management. Many Trusts will employ specialist midwives to care for a defined group of women with particular needs, for example a teen-age pregnancy or bereavement midwife. A fairly recent development in the NHS is the position of Consultant Midwife; the majority of Trusts are now fortunate to have such a senior midwife who is able to provide leadership and foster excellence in clinical practice.

Many candidates seeking a career in midwifery will have clear ideas of what they think the role entails – most people will perceive that role within the labour ward, supporting women to birth their babies. However, childbirth is a continuum that means that the birth of a baby is only one part of the journey to becoming a mother. This is impor-tant to consider as Admissions tutors will tell you that many candidates have a very idealised vision of midwifery practice, and fail to grasp that the realities of the role can be light years away from perceived expectations.

During the 1980s when I trained first to be a nurse, then a midwife, the NHS seemed a far simpler place, with less demands on the service and the carers within it. Partly, this perceived simplicity can be related to the different expectations of healthcare consumers, and partly by the way the organisation was run at that time. For example, each ward had its own team of domestic staff, rather than the current contractual system where the staff can change frequently. The importance of consumerism hadn't yet made a significant impact on the NHS, and many areas of prac-tice had not evolved much in a number of years. We take it for granted now that keyhole surgery is the 'norm' for many procedures, enabling swift recovery and a reduced hospital stay, yet this is a relatively recent development – in 1984, the removal of a gall bladder necessitated at least a week in hospital. Similarly, women today with complex health needs can successfully and safely give birth – in 1988, it was extremely rare to care for a woman in labour who was HIV positive, or who had conceived through assisted reproduction techniques, unless you worked in major units. Now both of these are relatively commonplace.

Midwives and nurses have subsequently seen major changes both to their role, and to the NHS itself. This is essentially the driver for an all-graduate profession. Generally, the concept of 'graduateness' encompasses a range of attributes and abilities that are required of a dynamic, complex profession. These include leadership, responsiveness and the ability to question existing practice. Given some of the changes already described here, perhaps you can start to see why the midwife of the future must have a more sophisticated 'tool kit' of skills in order to continue to provide the excellent care women deserve, and respond to the changing health needs of society. The majority of midwifery students have completed degree courses for some time now, although it is difficult to quantify the impact that graduate midwives have made yet as the variables are complex. You can read about the impending move to an all-graduate nursing profession in the next section.

As part of the research that you are required to do before you apply, and therefore to ensure that you choose the right profession, it is vitally important that you become more familiar with some of these issues in order to strengthen your application. This is also to be absolutely sure that you know what you're letting yourself in for! For midwifery, a key document to read and absorb is *Midwifery 2020*, a government report that sets out to identify how midwifery care can be maximised to meet the changing needs of women and their families. A link to this document is provided in the Further Reading section at the end of the chapter. At this point, you may be wondering why such a document is needed. You would be right to observe, for example, that the usual way women give birth hasn't changed since we started walking upright, or that women still require midwives who are kind, empathetic and supportive to care for them. However, the needs of women and their families have become more complex over the years and subsequently demand an expansion of the core skills already mentioned. For example, as a student midwife, I was not expected to routinely screen women for domestic abuse, yet this is now a 'standard' enquiry during pregnancy. Domestic abuse is not a new phenomenon, rather our understanding of the causes and effects is becoming more widely understood. The implications for midwives and women of such developments are therefore highly significant and demand skills and abilities that impact on midwifery education, research and practice. In short, women and midwives haven't changed, however the political and cultural landscape where childbirth occurs is no longer the same.

Many candidates struggle to differentiate between the professions, and find the differences between nursing and midwifery to be somewhat blurred. Hopefully, this section has now begun to answer that question, as will reading the suggested resources. From professional experience, the essential difference perhaps lies within the nature and expectations of the healthcare consumers themselves. Thus, most women experiencing childbirth will be healthy and require a different sort of care from that required by a patient recovering from major surgery or illness – the expectations, priorities and experiences of the consumers are very different and therefore demand very different skills. However, they both still expect, need and deserve **care**. This is the fundamental principle within nursing and midwifery – how this principle specifically applies within the professions will be explored further throughout this book.

Nursing specifics

Jo Rouse

Nurse education, like midwifery, is based in universities and while you will spend half of your time in a university learning the knowledge and skills that underpin nursing, the remaining half of your time will be in practice learning placements, where you will use your knowledge and skills to deliver nursing care directly to patients. Universities, NHS Trusts and other organisations both within the NHS and the private sector work very closely together in partnership to deliver high-quality education.

On successful completion of initial nurse education, nurses gain both registration with the Nursing and Midwifery Council (NMC) that enables nurses to obtain employment as a staff nurse, and an academic award. This award has been at least a Diploma in Higher Education, which is equivalent to two-thirds of a degree. Some students have chosen to continue their studies and obtain a degree in nursing.

However, in order to prepare for the future and to make sure that nurses will be able to meet the changing needs of adults and children in the years to come, the NMC have extensively reviewed the existing provision of nurse education. This review has involved consultation with patients, service users and carers, as well as qualified nurses, NHS Trusts and universities about how nurse education is delivered. The results mean two changes for nurse education. Firstly, although nurses must have specialised knowledge and skills to care for particular groups of people, now called **fields of practice** - **Adults**, adults with **Learning Disabilities** or **Mental Health** needs and **Children** - nurses must have the basic **generic** knowledge and skills to provide nursing care for any patient or client. Secondly, the number of graduate nurses has already been increasing over recent years, and now that teaching all nursing students to degree level will be introduced, the associated skills required should advance nursing practice. For example, graduate nurses will be able to think critically in different and complicated situations and be able to analyse and to solve problems at a higher level.

So, while your nurse education will still take three years and will still mean that you spend half of your time in university and half of your time in placement giving direct patient care, you will now learn generic nursing skills and knowledge as well as field of practice specific skills and knowledge. Generic skills and knowledge are those which all nurses, irrespective of their field of practice, must be able to apply, and field of practice specific skills and knowledge relate specifically to those required for that field. To be successful in nurse education, the generic and field of practice specific skills and knowledge you will need to demonstrate competence in are divided into four areas called domains. These are: **professional values, communication and interpersonal skills, nursing practice and decision-making** and finally, **leadership, management and team working**. More information about these domains is available on the NMC website (www.nmc-uk.org).

Your nursing programme will normally be divided into three equal parts, with each part being separated by a progression point. The NMC have identified specific knowledge, skills and attributes that you will need to be able to demonstrate at each progression point before you can move on to the next stage of your education. The NMC suggest that the requirements at these progression points will depend on how a particular university arranges practice placements within their programme as well as reflecting the knowledge, skills and attributes that are considered important by the practice placements.

Examples of the knowledge, skills and attributes required at each progression point relate to ensuring the safety of your patients and clients, their carers and families, as well as professional values, attitudes and behaviours that must be shown towards all people, their carers, families and the people you will work with. As you progress through the programme, you will need to demonstrate that you can achieve these whilst working more independently and with less supervision, safely and with increasing confidence. This means that as you start your nurse education, you will be given a lot of support, supervision and guidance to help you to learn these new skills and attributes and to help you to increase your confidence and competence. By the end of your education, as you register as a nurse with the NMC, you will be able to practise all of the required skills and attributes confidently and autonomously.

Students undertaking nurse education have benefited from a NHS bursary which covers the cost of tuition fees and in some cases, gives the students a monthly income to help meet their living and studying expenses. The bursary is different from a student loan because the bursary is yours to keep, whereas a loan must eventually be paid back! The bursary scheme is currently being reviewed by the Department of Health. To keep up to date with any changes that may be made to the scheme, you can read more on the Department of Health website (http://www.dh.gov.uk/).

The changes to an all-graduate nursing profession will take place over the next few years and will be completed by 2013. This means that some universities will be offering nurse education at Diploma in Higher Education as well as Degree level for a while longer, whereas some universities will only now offer Degree level nurse education. New entrants for nursing at the University of Worcester, for example, will only be offered graduate level education from September 2011.

The decision to do a degree or a diploma is a very individual one and will depend on the qualifications you have and where you want to study. However, there are many qualified nurses who are educated to diploma level (diplomats as opposed to graduates) and are really excellent nurses. Diplomats have the opportunity to 'top up' their diploma to a degree by completing further study at university.

Yvonne

Yvonne registered as an adult nurse with a Diploma in Higher Education 18 months ago. Since registering, Yvonne has been working as a staff nurse on a medical ward. Yvonne has had lots of opportunities to practise and further develop the skills and knowledge she learned during her nurse education. With the support of her colleagues, she quickly increased her confidence as a staff nurse and felt able to take responsibility for being in charge of her ward during her shifts. Recently, Yvonne has decided that she wants to continue her professional development and, in the future, would like to become a ward sister. To achieve her ambition, Yvonne has decided to return to university to 'top up' her diploma and get a degree. Because Yvonne wants to continue to work while studying, she will study on a part-time basis and aims to complete her degree in two years' time.

Case study 1.1

Sally

Sally registered as a children's nurse with a degree at the same time as Yvonne. However, Sally has been working as a staff nurse on a children's ward. Sally was also able to practise the skills and knowledge she learned during her nurse education and has decided to specialise in children's respiratory nursing. Sally successfully applied for a specialist nurse post as a junior sister and has decided to return to university to further her professional development and increase her knowledge and skills required as a specialist nurse. Sally has decided to start her Masters degree and to enable her to continue to work will complete this on a part-time basis over two years.

Case study 1.2

The move to all-graduate nursing does mean changes to the entry requirements universities will ask for and these will vary between universities. You can find out exactly what the entry requirements are for your chosen universities by looking on their website or by using the University and College Application Service (UCAS) website (**http://www .ucas.ac.uk/**). You can also look at the examples of university courses provided in Chapter 2.

In addition to the stated academic entry requirements, the NMC also set some additional requirements for nursing, similar to those they set for midwifery. Some of these are academic requirements, for example related to the level of English, Maths and Information Technology you must be able to evidence when you apply. Other requirements are associated with 'Good health and Good character'. Again, you can read more about this on the university and NMC websites before you start your nurse education.

There is a huge difference between caring and nursing and you must be sure this difference is understood before you apply. While caring and compassion are vital attributes for nurses, providing nursing care is different from providing social care. Nurses focus on the needs of the individual, rather than specific illnesses or conditions. They help individuals and their families to live more comfortable lives by providing nursing care that sometimes requires invasive procedures to be performed, with consent. This care also involves the use of medical technology, pharmacology and information technology as well as providing advice and counselling. You will need to demonstrate that you really do understand the role of a nurse and what a nurse actually does to be successful in your application and selection for nurse education. If you don't have any experience working in the healthcare sector, the best place to start is by reading. You can access books and relevant journals through your local library, or subscribe to nursing journals, although this will incur a cost.

To summarise briefly:

- In **Adult** nursing, you will care for any adult from age 18 years through to care of the older person with diverse health requirements, including acute or long-term illnesses, as well as providing advice and support to adults to enable them to remain healthy. You will work as a staff nurse in hospitals or the community – in people's homes, in health centres or in nursing homes both within the NHS and private sectors. You will work closely with patients and members of the multi-disciplinary team (doctors, physiotherapists,

occupational therapists, pharmacists, radiographers etc.) to provide holistic care. Your nurse education will enable you to assess,
plan, implement and evaluate care for individual patients.

- **Learning disability** nurses work in partnership with individuals,
  their families and carers and other professionals to support the
  well-being and social inclusion of people with learning disabilities.
  Essential aspects of this include removing barriers and reducing
  stigma as well as maintaining physical and mental health. Again,
  the settings that learning disabilities nurses work in vary from
  residential homes to working in the individual's home or even
  workplaces.

- Most mentally ill patients and clients are nursed in the community rather than hospital settings. The range of **mental health**
  conditions is vast and as a mental health nurse you will need to
  use effective communication and interpersonal skills to develop
  therapeutic relationships with your clients and their families.
  Multi-agency working is also an important factor, as you will be
  working with psychiatrists, social workers, therapists and carers.

- **Children** have varying needs as they develop from infancy to child-
  hood, adolescence and to adulthood. As a children's nurse you will
  develop skills to communicate with children of all ages and abilities.
  You will develop skills and knowledge to keep children healthy as
  well as those to reduce the impact of physical and mental illness
  and disease. Working with the parents or child's carers is an essential part of this role. You will work in a variety of settings including
  hospitals, schools, GP surgeries and health centres and of course, the
  child's home. It might be timely to return now to the reflections/
  diaries of nurses offered earlier in this chapter.

Summary

- **Nursing and midwifery together are one of the top five most popular
  courses for UCAS applications.**

- **Understanding the key differences between nursing and midwifery
  is vital to successful application and helps ensure that candidates
  embark on the right career path.**

- The key skills and attributes of nurses and midwives include communication, compassion, empathy, patience and caring.

- Nursing is primarily concerned with the care of individuals with diverse health requirements, including acute and chronic illness, as well as the provision of advice and support for those individuals to remain healthy. This involves planning, implementing and evaluating care for individual patients.

- Midwifery is primarily focused on the care and support of women during normal pregnancy, birth and early motherhood, including the promotion of breastfeeding. Midwives also recognise and act when childbirth becomes complicated in order to ensure maternal and neonatal well-being.

- Nursing and midwifery demand a range of high-order skills if the complex nature of changing healthcare needs are to be fully met. These include leadership, decision-making and responsiveness.

- The majority of pre-registration midwifery courses have been at degree level for a number of years.

- The impact of graduate midwives on the experiences of women and midwives is not yet fully established.

- Nursing is rapidly moving towards being an all-graduate profession.

Further reading

Ehrenreich B, English D. *Witches, Midwives and Nurses: A History of Women Healers*. Available at: www.tmh.floonet.net/articles/witches.html

Midwifery 2020: Delivering expectations. Available at: www.midwifery2020.org

Nursing and Midwifery Council. See: www.nmc-uk.org

Royal College of Midwives. See: www.rcm.org.uk

Royal College of Nursing. See: www.rcn.org.uk

UK Centre for the History of Nursing and Midwifery. See: www.nursing.manchester.ac.uk/ukchnm/aboutus

Chapter 2

Starting the journey

Learning outcomes

By the end of Chapter 2, you should be able to:

- ✔ appreciate the range of entry routes available, for example the Access Diploma, and make an informed choice in the context of your own circumstances
- ✔ review examples of university nursing and midwifery course academic entry requirements
- ✔ consider some of the 'selling' points universities offer to help you choose the right location
- ✔ utilise the provided checklist tool to help summarise the strengths and weaknesses of various universities during open/visit days

Introduction

This chapter explores the application journey that candidates take along the road to professionalisation. Firstly, it will consider some of the entry routes candidates negotiate along this journey. Some examples of the range of university courses on offer are then provided in order to demonstrate the range of entry criteria demanded. As a vital part of this process involves the selection of the best university for you, an open day checklist is provided for use during the various visits that you will make to university campuses throughout the UK. Although the content of nursing and midwifery courses has to follow a similar format determined by the NMC, the delivery of that content, the learning and teaching strategies, and the quality of the student experience will all vary enormously. The checklist will therefore be an invaluable tool to aid your recall and ultimately make the right choice.

Entry routes

The increased popularity of nursing and midwifery programmes has driven the entry criteria demanded by institutions higher each year. As part of your decision-making process, for example thinking that it would be nice to complete a nursing degree by the seaside, or a midwifery programme in an area with a high homebirth rate, you need to be aware that entry criteria vary between universities, even ones within the same geographical area. Examples of the range of criteria will be provided in this chapter. However, the key point for you to remember here is to check the entry criteria *before* you apply, and don't rely on local knowledge to predict what is required elsewhere.

The NMC make broad recommendations regarding the academic qualifications required for consideration of a place on a nursing or midwifery undergraduate programme. However, universities have the right to adapt this basic level and set their own criteria. Entry requirements will therefore depend on demand and supply. An increase in applications to courses tends to drive entry criteria higher in tandem, although the widening participation agenda does also influence universities in moderating their response in order to ensure that non-traditional applicants are not unfairly disadvantaged.

Universities generally operate within the UCAS tariff points system – level 3 qualifications such as 'A' levels, Diplomas and Certificates are given a numerical value that adds up to the candidate's overall points package. You can view the tariff tables at www.ucas.com. Traditional students, that is young people doing 'A' levels, will be fairly familiar with UCAS points as each grade at 'A' level equates to different points; an A grade = 100 points; B grade = 80 points; C grade = 60 points etc. Where a university course demands 240 UCAS points for example, a typical offer may be based on something like BBB. Universities will also demand a package of GCSEs, often including Maths, English and Science.

Although this is fairly straightforward for 'A' level students, do remember to check the entry criteria very carefully, especially when considering several different institutions. For example, certain relevant subjects may also be required, such as a science or social science. If you were reading an applicant's personal statement to join a nursing course and their 'A' levels included highly specialised subjects such as photography or art history, what would you think about their motivation and interest in nursing? Of course, we all make wrong choices in life and this candidate could still succeed, especially if s/he follows some of the suggestions to be found later in this book.

For non-traditional students, the picture can be more complicated. The requirement to achieve a certain level of qualifications before even starting a nursing or midwifery course can be bewildering and alarming, especially if you have been out of education for some time. Some of these concerns are addressed in Chapter 5 and the suggestions there should go some way to allaying these anxieties. Perhaps the biggest concern for non-traditional candidates is that they will be alone in a group of younger women/men who have all followed the usual 'A' level route. Well, you might be reassured to know that cohort groups of student midwives and nurses encompass a broad range of academic background and therefore age range. To illustrate this, have a look at the age/entry qualification profiles of recent cohorts of student nurses and midwives at Worcester shown in Tables 2.1-2.4.

Table 2.1 Entry qualifications of pre-registration nursing students

Qualification	Number of students
PG dip/PG cert	4
First degree	29
Higher national certificate (HNC)	1
'A' levels	15
BTEC	6
Access to Higher Education Diploma	4
NVQ 3	28
Other	4

Table 2.2 Entry qualifications of pre-registration midwifery students

Qualification	Number of students
First degree	4
'A' levels	6
BTEC	2
Access to Higher Education Diploma	8
Other	2

Table 2.3 Age ranges of pre-registration nursing students

Age range	Number of students
18-25	44
25-40	34
40+	14

**Table 2.4   Age ranges of pre-registration
midwifery students**

Age range	Number of students
18-25	9
25-40	13
40+	-

Access and BTEC Diplomas are examples of equivalent level 3 qualifications, i.e. for those people who don't have 'A' levels, or may not have been in formal education for some years. Most further education colleges, often on a part-time basis, offer these programmes and they may also be financially subsidised. The content can be intense and assessment load demanding. However, many midwifery and nursing candidates state that these programmes helped them significantly, both in terms of refreshing study skills, and by providing opportunities to study relevant subjects. In the same way that universities demand different UCAS points, be aware that this has echoes with the Access Diploma. For example, different institutions may require different quantities of overall merits and distinctions, and demand that additional modules be studied if candidates do not have a suitable 'package' of GCSE qualifications. BTEC is usually more straightforward as the level of award corresponds to the UCAS points system – see the UCAS tariff tables for more detailed information **www.ucas.com**. However, be aware that some universities do ask for a higher level of award with BTEC so ensure that you do thorough research *before* you apply.

It is also possible to study the Access Diploma via the distance learning route and this may be an attractive pathway for some candidates. For example, this might suit if your lifestyle doesn't support regular attendance at a college, or you live in a geographically isolated part of the world. This style of study can be a lonely experience and demands a high level of motivation and commitment from the learner. However, even when it isn't face-to-face, the encouragement and support from tutors makes all the difference to a student's experience of learning, and you would therefore be wise to find out in advance what type/frequency/regularity of support is included in the distance learning package before you commit. My general advice is to ask yourself this key question – are you the type of person who can consistently study independently, or do you need a nudge from regular interaction with other students and tutors? For further information, see the Distance Learning Centre's website (http://www.distance-learning-centre.co.uk).

 ## Examples of university courses

Now that you have worked, or are working towards the academic entry requirements, and are clear about what it is you actually want to become, you now need to choose universities that offer a nursing or midwifery programme that suits you best. Remember that if you successfully complete a programme, all universities will enable you to register with the NMC as a nurse or midwife, plus award a degree/diploma. The key factors influencing your decision are therefore related to *how* the university delivers its programmes, together with *where* you want to live and work for three years.

The NMC set out minimum standards for pre-registration nursing and midwifery, and these standards shape curriculum development at each university. The standards can be viewed at the NMC's website (www .nmc-uk.org). However, just as universities can adopt their own entry criteria, they can also incorporate the NMC guidelines in a flexible way. For example, all student midwives have to spend a proportion of their clinical placements based within the community setting – where those placements occur during a programme will vary between universities and is dependent on a number of issues, such as student numbers and geographical location. If you have not yet passed your driving test for example, it may be more practical for you to select universities whose community placements are well served by public transport, or don't occur until the latter half of the first year, thus allowing you time to pass your test.

So, clinical placements all vary between universities, as do the number of students in a cohort group, the types of learning opportunities available, and the flexibility of the programme itself. Some universities offer graduates a 'fast track' route into nursing, for example, and you can read about one example of this type of programme later on in this chapter (see University Example 2.7). Don't forget to look for hidden costs such as how much bus fare you will need travelling to your community base, or car parking charges when you are able to travel independently. A major cost for students living away from home is accommodation rental charges and all this needs to be taken into account before you commit to your chosen university. In Chapter 5, you will read about one student's strategy for keeping her costs to a minimum.

It is therefore very important that you get to know your chosen university and the nursing or midwifery programme offered well in advance. All universities will have websites that provide a good indication of what's on offer, but probably the best way to inform your decision-making is to go along to a university open day. There, you will have an opportunity to meet teaching staff and students, ask questions, tour the campus, view accommodation packages and get a 'feel' for the surrounding location. The atmosphere generated by a busy inner city university will be very different from one that has a campus some miles from the centre, and this may be important to you and the overall experience you're seeking to achieve. Remember that you're about to invest three years of your life in this unfamiliar environment, so take your time to come to a decision.

Competition for over-subscribed courses, such as child health nursing or midwifery, will necessitate application to several universities in order to maximise the chance of success. As numerous visits to different institutions can quickly become a blur, a checklist has been provided at the end of this chapter (see pp. 50–51), designed to be completed during the various open days that you attend. It may help jog your memory of the various universities visited, as well as be a useful summary to aid the decision-making process.

To help you further, there now follow some examples of nursing and midwifery courses on offer at a variety of different universities. These have been included to demonstrate the variety of entry requirements and courses on offer, not to suggest that one university is 'better' than another. Please note that the stated entry requirements may no longer be up to date and therefore you *must* check directly with the institution, or via the UCAS website (**www.ucas.com**).

University Example 2.1
Edge Hill University (Midwifery)

(www.edgehill.ac.uk)

This course requires 280 UCAS points (or equivalent), plus 5 GCSEs at grade C or above, including English Language and Mathematics, and evidence of academic study in the previous five years.

The programme comprises approximately 50 per cent practice and 50 per cent theory, both of which are assessed and contribute to the final degree classification. Each year of the programme has its own specific theme and contains a module, which introduces and develops understanding of interprofessional disciplines and multi-professional working. All modules in the midwifery programme are compulsory.

The first year focuses on normal pregnancy, with learning centred on the effect pregnancy has on physiology and how this is applied to clinical practice. In the second year students study the pathophysiology of pregnancy related conditions and implement this knowledge in clinical practice. The third and final year of the programme not only consolidates the knowledge and understanding acquired in years one and two, but enables students to develop their interest in a chosen area of midwifery, or related practice. To achieve this students engage in a self-funded, elective placement, which may be undertaken either locally, nationally or internationally. This module directly responds to the UK's increasingly diverse multi-racial and multi-cultural society, which requires midwives to work in maternity services that meet the need for ethically sound and culturally sensitive care. Students also engage with a small, supervised caseload of women for whom they provide bespoke, holistic, continuous care throughout the pregnancy continuum, which includes on-calls to attend labour and birth.

A strong grounding in evidence-based practice coupled with a dynamic and innovative curriculum that address the demands of a constantly evolving service produces highly employable, professionally competent graduate midwives who are fit for practice, purpose and award. The university is one of the top ten for graduate employment, which in relation to midwifery may, in part, be due to the structure of the practice element of the programme exposing the students to diverse models of midwifery care. This is evidenced through every student having to engage in:

- a range of clinical placements in all of our three provider NHS Trusts;
- carrying a small, supervised caseload of women for whom they provide continuous care throughout the pregnancy continuum, including on-calls for support during labour and birth;
- an elective placement in a local, national or international maternity or maternity related setting.

Consequently Edge Hill University produces students who, at the point of qualification, are rigorously prepared for both autonomous practice and independent practice; are able to meet the needs and requirements of the women and families they care for in the context of the UK's developing multi-racial and multi-cultural society, and who are also able to respond to the government's agenda for service delivery.

Further support for the strength of our programme can be evidenced from the commendations received at the recent validation of a new programme (April 2010) for two of the modules that contribute to the above. We also have a robust admissions process, for which we were again commended by the validating panel.

Jane Knibbs, Midwifery Lecturer

University Example 2.2
University Campus Suffolk (Midwifery)

(www.ucs.ac.uk)

University Campus Suffolk (UCS) invites potential applicants with 240 UCAS tariff points to include GCSEs in English, Mathematics and Science to apply for the BSc (Hons) Midwifery.

Studying midwifery combines theory studies at the new state-of-the-art campus waterfront buildings and practice in one of three NHS Trust hospitals across Suffolk and South Norfolk. The course supports students to develop a range of knowledge, skills and competencies in accordance with the Nursing and Midwifery Council (NMC) Standards.

Teaching combines a range of face-to-face sessions, some large lecture groups, smaller group sessions, discussions and group presentations aimed to stimulate students' interests and a range of learning styles. These sessions are supported by individual and group work on the University Virtual Learning Environment and by practical sessions in the Skills Laboratory. There are excellent links between the students, lecturers and midwives in practice; currently the students, their practice mentor and personal tutor, meet at least twice a year, to assess and develop a personal plan for each student.

The range of assessments is innovative and allows each student to develop their creative as well as academic skills, including poster presentations, reflections from practice, a portfolio, as well as assignments, a dissertation, one oral and one written exam. For each assessment a personal tutor and module leader will support the student to reach their potential.

UCS currently offer extra curricula activities such as a midwifery book club, to read and discuss books suggested by student midwives that are novels, autobiographies or other resources relevant to your studies. For the less avid reader plans are afoot for a film club, to discuss representations of women, childbirth and the family in traditional and contemporary media formats.

Sam Chenery-Morris, Senior Lecturer

University Example 2.3
Birmingham City University (Child Health Nursing)

(www.bcu.ac.uk/health)

Birmingham City University (BCU) has a long tradition of training children's nurses and has made a significant contribution to the National Health Service workforce supporting children and young people's healthcare needs. BCU offers two routes of entry into pre-registration nurse training:

1. Three-year BSc (Hons) Nursing RN course – two intakes per year, April and September (Course Code B730).
2. Two-year Graduate Diploma course – one intake per year in April (Course Code 3310).

Children's nursing demands a variety of skills and attributes, which includes the achievement of course specific entry requirements. The following table summarises our entry requirements – further details are available on the UCAS website (**www.ucas.com**) and our university institution code is B25.

BSc (Hons) Nursing RN Entry Requirements – Course Code B730	Graduate Diploma Entry Requirements – Course Code 3310
Level 2 qualifications must be achieved prior to application. GCSE at Grade C or above in five subjects and must include English Language, Mathematics and a Science.	Level 2 qualifications must be achieved prior to application. GCSE in English Language at Grade C or above (if Degree not taught and assessed in English Language) and Grade C in Mathematics.
Other acceptable qualifications include:	GCSE equivalents *not* acceptable. Plus:
· a minimum of 240 UCAS tariff points · 'A' levels · BTEC Nationals · Level 3 Access Course · other comparable qualifications.	· First Degree minimum grade 2:2 · AS level with relevant content and experience i.e. Sociology, Psychology · AP(E)L minimum of 550 hours' practical experience relevant to nursing.

Strengths of studying at BCU include the opportunity to engage in e-learning, which is risk-free, utilising state-of-the-art technology such as virtual cases, simulation and immersive clinical environments while developing hands-on clinical skills in the world-famous Birmingham Children's Hospital.

Cathy Poole, Senior Lecturer in Child Health/Admissions Tutor

University Example 2.4
Northumbria University (Nursing and Midwifery)

(www.northumbria.ac.uk)

The five branches of nursing available are:

- Adult (280 points);
- Mental Health (280 points);
- Child (280 points);
- Learning Disability (280 points);
- Midwifery BSc programme (280 points).

As a minimum requirement students are also required to have passes in Mathematics, English and a science subject.

At Northumbria we offer a progressive and dynamic curriculum. It prepares students from all branches of nursing and midwifery to deliver high-quality care to meet the needs of patients in the twenty-first century.

Throughout the programme we use a variety of teaching, learning and assessment strategies. We have lectures, seminars and practical sessions, guided study time, exams, assignments and presentations. Placements range from six weeks to twenty-one weeks and are to a variety of clinical areas, both hospital and community based. Some students are allocated a 'home' NHS Trust while others are located within a geographical area.

Clinical skills are taught and developed in our newly expanded Clinical Skills Centre. We have a wide range of equipment to allow our students to develop their skills and knowledge in an innovative, interactive and controlled environment prior to going into clinical placements. We have developed simulation of practice to be used at a very basic level to develop psychomotor skills, for example, learning to take pulse and blood pressure, to managing a critically ill patient to develop clinical reasoning and decision-making skills. Simulation exercises are done as an individual or in groups depending on the learning outcomes of the modules.

We have excellent IT and library facilities within the university, and students will be expected to use our electronic platform for learning from the beginning of the course. Module information can be downloaded from the e-learning platform.

Fiona M Adair, Senior Lecturer Adult Nursing/Admissions Tutor

---

University Example 2.5
Oxford Brookes University (Nursing and Midwifery)

(www.brookes.ac.uk)

The Oxford hospitals have been providing professional healthcare education since the 1920s and now in partnership with Oxford Brookes University have an excellent and consistent reputation for offering a welcoming and supportive environment in which to learn. Oxford Brookes University offers undergraduate and postgraduate nursing (adult, children's and mental heath) and midwifery degree courses, and also provides interdisciplinary focused pre-qualification courses in Health and Social Care, Occupational Therapy, Osteopathy, Operating Department Practice, Paramedic Emergency Care, Physiotherapy, and Social Work.

Practice education is central to all our courses and we offer an extensive range of placement settings, all of which have excellent reputations for the quality of their clinical services. The emphasis throughout our courses is on practice-based learning and skills development, underpinned by a relevant and contemporary knowledge base.

We have an excellent track record of high levels of student satisfaction, low student attrition rates and high employability. Teaching is facilitated by our specialist subject lecturers and includes practice partners and service users. A number of the academic staff also hold clinically based posts alongside their teaching responsibilities.

Achieving a high quality student experience is a key commitment for Oxford Brookes. Students, external examiners and reviewers also regularly commend course teams for the outstanding support and advice given to students throughout their time here.

Entry requirements for Nursing and Midwifery Degree courses are typically three 'A' Levels, as follows:

- Adult Nursing – grades CCC (science preferred) or equivalent;
- Children's Nursing – grades BBC with at least one science subject, or equivalent vocational 'A' levels;
- Mental Health Nursing – grades CCC or equivalent;
- Midwifery (three-year and short course) – grades BBC including at least one science subject (i.e. Chemistry or Biology), or equivalent vocational 'A' levels.

Come and see us and find out more. We hold regular open days throughout the year; for details, go to: **http://shsc.brookes.ac.uk/opendays**

We would be really pleased to meet you.

Juliet Bostwick, Programme Leader Adult Nursing Course

University Example 2.6
University of Hertfordshire (Nursing)

(www.herts.ac.uk)

The University of Hatfield School of Nursing, Midwifery and Social Work offers courses in pre-registration nursing. To gain a place on a course, students require the following:

- Five GCSEs grade C or above to include English and Mathematics;
- UCAS tariff points: 240 from at least two 'A' levels or other equivalent qualifications;
- Access to Higher Education (Nursing) course 45 level 3 credits of which at least 24 must be merits.

Nursing at the University of Hertfordshire provides a challenging but dynamic course, which focuses on ensuring our students are prepared to enter the changing and exciting world of healthcare as qualified practitioners. Practical skills are taught in designated laboratories, including a recently furbished child specific one; this provides a safe environment for the practise and acquisition of practical skills. Skills will encompass a full and comprehensive range from learning to take a patient's temperature to managing the simulated ward. Students will have opportunities to develop critical, analytical and reflective skills that will enable them to make sound judgements and provide high-quality nursing care. Confidence with practical skills underpinned with relevant and evidenced-based theory will allow students to undertake their practice placements with a sound knowledge base. University-based study days are interspersed with clinical practice; these will include acute hospital settings and a large variety of community and non-NHS placements. Students have an opportunity to choose their own elective placement at the end of year two, enabling them to experience nursing in a different context, either in the UK or abroad. Students qualifying from the University of Hertfordshire have excellent job opportunities in the local area, London and further afield.

The University of Hertfordshire has a range of excellent facilities including a 24-hour learning resource centre, state-of-the-art sports facilities, modern accommodation and a new Health Research building with a range of health simulation opportunities. The new student Forum venue incorporates a night club, three bars and food outlets and Hatfield itself is only 20 minutes from central London.

Sheila Roberts, Senior Lecturer/Admissions Tutor

University Example 2.7
University of Nottingham (Derby Centre) (Nursing)

(http://pgstudy.nottingham.ac.uk)

The Postgraduate Diploma (PGDip) in Nursing Studies provides the opportunity for those with a first degree and an interest in pursuing nursing as a career to undertake an accelerated two-year full-time programme of study. In addition to the academic qualification of a postgraduate diploma, the course leads to a Nursing and Midwifery Council (NMC) recognised professional qualification and registration in *either* Adult, Mental Health or Children's nursing. On completion there is the option of further study to complete an MSc in Nursing Studies.

The course itself is divided equally between taught theory and clinical experience across a range of healthcare settings. The course has been commended by the NMC for the quality of its learning, for embracing a partnership approach to educational provision and for the involvement of service users and carers within the programme. The University of Nottingham consistently scores highly in respect of its nursing educational provision and was rated as one of the top five places to study nursing within the UK in the *Guardian* Newspaper's Best University Guide 2009.

Course innovations include: interprofessional learning with medical students, the opportunity to explore other healthcare systems and health cultures through an international 'buddy', a problem-based learning curriculum in which students identify their own learning needs through real-life video scenarios, and a clinical adviser for second-year students to aid career progression.

Entry requirements are as follows:

- Honours Degree 2:2 or above;
- minimum of five GCSEs including English and Mathematics at grade C or above;
- candidates have to be citizens of the EU.

Susan Thompson, Deputy Director, Graduate Entry Nursing

 ## 'But I'm still not sure'

Ideally, after you've done your background reading, visited so many universities that your head is spinning, and reflected on the knowledge acquired so far, you'll be in a good position to not only apply, but also feel confident in your choice of profession or field of practice. However, many candidates are still unsure at this stage and can quickly lose sight of their goal. This self-doubt can be very disconcerting for candidates and this is when an Admissions tutor can become your best friend. Remember that s/he will have spent many years working in clinical practice before moving into higher education, and therefore has a rich pot of expertise to utilise in the provision of relevant information.

However, do remember that part of the role of the Admissions tutor is to advise and provide appropriate information, not to do your background work or make the ultimate decision for you. There are perhaps two paths to now consider.

Be honest with yourself about the reasons for being unsure and perhaps defer your application until you have found out more, for example by obtaining a position as a healthcare assistant that will give you an excellent and very realistic taste of the clinical world. It's difficult to imagine how exhausting night shifts can be, or how challenging some aspects of practice are unless you actually engage with that alien world. Sometimes, people struggle at this point because they have doubts that nursing or midwifery is really the right choice for them, at this particular stage of their life. It's perfectly acceptable to have these doubts – not everyone can rise to the demands of practice where your acts (or omissions) can change the course of someone's life for ever.

Find out if your preferred universities offer any type of programme/ event that helps illuminate some of these realities and book yourself onto it. One such innovation has been pioneered at Worcester and is known as the Midwifery Taster Day (MTD). It was born in 2002 after an easy gestation, although as the initiative grows older, further challenges present themselves. I moved into higher education in 2001 and was quickly struck by the lack of realism displayed by midwifery candidates at interview. Understanding full well the demands of practice and the skills required of midwifery students as they negotiate these demands, led me to develop an initiative that would give candidates seeking a midwifery career a 'taste' of midwifery.

The key strength of the MTD lies with the involvement of current midwifery students – part of day involves them leading practical workshops that involve the use of equipment that simulates normal birth and antenatal examination, amongst others. The workshops showcase the skills required of midwifery students early on in the course, as well as provide an opportunity to find out the absolute truth about a midwifery course. I know, because the students tell me, that they are extremely frank with taster day attendees about some of the difficulties they encounter along the way, such as financial, assessment or relationship crises.

The MTD has been adopted by other colleagues within the university, and it is consistently recognised by the NMC as an example of good Admissions practice. Other universities have taken the initiative one step further, for example by offering candidates a brief clinical placement before they commit to a midwifery programme (McIntyre, 2011). You would be wise, therefore, to investigate any type of initiative that serves to illuminate the realities of practice/student life. However, one note of caution – my experience has shown that such programmes can actually be counterproductive for some candidates who have a persistently 'starry eyed' approach to midwifery. For example, they witness accomplished student midwives performing simulated skills with ease and confidence, without adequately reflecting on the time, effort or compromise that the student has invested as part of his/her learning curve. So, by all means attend such events, but remember that they are just one small step in your journey and to leave your rose-tinted spectacles behind!

Summary

- Candidates for nursing and midwifery courses enter via a range of traditional ('A' levels) and non-traditional (Access) routes. Student nurse/midwife cohort groups are typically made up of people from a broad range of backgrounds. Universities welcome this demographic range as it enhances the student learning experience, and demonstrates that diversity is very important within healthcare.

- Academic entry requirements vary amongst universities and often increase each year. Candidates *must* check these on each individual institution's or the UCAS website *before* applying. Do not assume that institutions running the same programme of study will therefore have the same entry requirements.

- Make every effort to visit universities during dedicated open/taster events as these are an important step towards selecting the institution that best serves your individual learning needs. Remember that you are also researching your home for the next three years.

- Each university will have a unique selling point – be sure that you find out what it is.

- University visit days can quickly become a blur and by the time you reach home, you may have forgotten the key features of each one visited. To help avoid this trap, remember to complete the open day checklist provided at the end of this chapter.

- It's quite common to feel overwhelmed by the range and diversity of courses available and therefore perfectly acceptable, for example, to delay your application for a year. This time could be spent working within healthcare to obtain a completely realistic picture of your chosen profession, and provide some major clues as to your final destination. Far better to do this than commence a programme of study, only to leave fairly soon afterwards once reality kicks in and you discover that it isn't right for you after all.

Open day checklist

University	First impressions	Campus facilities	Accommodation	Location of clinical placements	Teaching and learning strategies	Course structure	University/ NHS Trusts relationship	Employment opportunities	Unique selling point

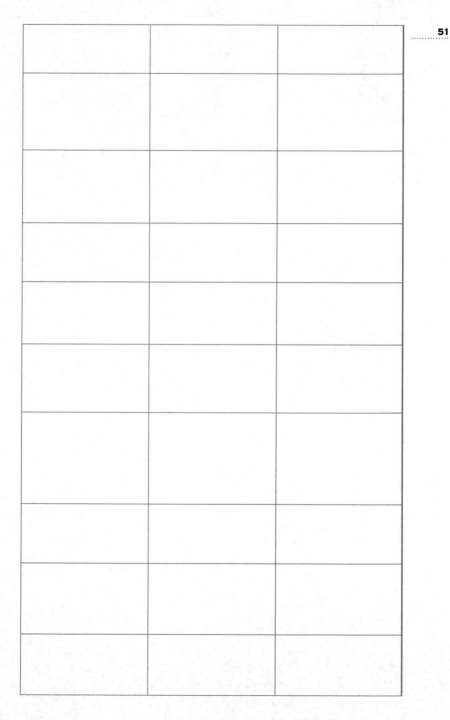

Chapter 3

Application and selection

Learning outcomes

By the end of Chapter 3, you should be able to:

✔ obtain structured advice about completing the UCAS application form and personal statement, guided by examples and suggestions drawn from practice

✔ understand the importance of accurately reflecting the field of nursing practice applied for

✔ appreciate the needs of applicants who have a disability, or past caution/conviction

✔ understand the rationale for the variety of selection day tasks candidates are expected to complete, and glean some top tips for success

✔ utilise the resources and tools provided to feel more confident when attending selection days

Introduction

This chapter focuses on application and selection, the goal that you have been working towards for months, or even years. A significant part of Chapter 3 looks at writing the personal statement, a task that can inspire terror in even the most optimistic candidate. If you have been 'rejected' at this stage before, you'll know at first hand that it is a complex task – how is it possible to 'sell' yourself in such a short number of permitted words? We then look at selection days, and an excellent range of advice and suggestions are provided to help prepare you for the next challenges that lie ahead on your journey. Neither of these stages are insurmountable – they just need lots of time and lots of effort.

 ## Completing the application form

All applications to nursing and midwifery programmes are made via UCAS each year during a predetermined application cycle that runs from mid-September to mid-January. Depending on the type of programme and locally determined commissioned places available, this application window may be rigorously enforced, i.e. applications may not be accepted outside the cycle. Remember that not all programmes engage with the 'clearing' process in August, especially those that are oversubscribed. Before you apply, it is necessary to first register with UCAS as either an individual applicant or via the school or college you are currently attending. The latter requires you to obtain the 'buzzword' from your school or college, used to complete the registration process.

For many candidates, the writing of the personal statement as part of the application process can provoke extreme stress and result in acute disappointment. However, when it is done well, the door to a healthcare course suddenly becomes wide open. The task cannot be completed quickly, or in isolation. It requires a high level of writing skill, yet should not be too formal. It must showcase a sophisticated understanding of the chosen profession, yet be written succinctly. It must show a clear rationale for choosing the profession, yet avoid being too personal. A task, therefore, not to be underestimated – yet it is not an impossible task to complete as long as some golden rules are followed. In order to illuminate these golden rules, it is useful to consider what makes a bad personal statement. I should add here that in my experience, the vast majority of candidates only submit 'bad' statements because they either have left it too late and struggled alone, or have not done enough research. The following pages focus on what causes a bad personal statement and how, instead, to write an effective personal statement.

Key misunderstandings of the profession

Thorough research before writing the personal statement (PS) should go a long way in preventing you from making a fundamental mistake about your chosen profession. For example, midwifery is not principally focused on the care and management of babies – it is a profession that chiefly supports *women* along all stages of the childbirth continuum. Although midwifery students are required to acquire detailed knowledge about infant feeding and care of the newborn in order to meet the required NMC standards, the focus is very much centred on the care and support of women. I have read a vast number of personal statements to the midwifery programme that confidently begin with something like:

I have wanted to be a midwife since obtaining work experience in a day nursery and really enjoy looking after babies and young children.

This can be a costly error and the likely rejection will cause huge disappointment. As well as Chapter 1 in this book, you would be wise to read extensively around the fundamental nature of your chosen profession; speak to relevant tutors at university open days and seek every opportunity to obtain helpful guidance and information. Excellent first starting points would be some or all of the websites listed in Chapter 1, for example the NMC (**www.nmc-uk.org**). These offer an extensive range of contemporary documents that afford a detailed view of the professions and should be key reading for applicants. In addition, Jo Rouse has already discussed some of these issues in the context of fields of practice in Chapter 1 and it would be good to review those now (see pp. 24-29). Jo discusses some further 'nursing specifics' to help with preparing your PS in Box 3.1.

Box 3.1 Nursing specifics

As part of your application to a nursing programme, you must demonstrate your knowledge and understanding of your chosen field of practice. You need to identify what skills and attributes you already possess that will support you in this field. If you have had relevant experience working in your field or with the public in general, you may be able to draw on that experience to give examples of the skills you have developed and why you consider them to be relevant. Remember, try not to list the work or placement experience you have had, but to explain what you learned from these experiences and how this will help you in learning to become a nurse in your chosen field of practice. Here is an example from an application form for adult nursing:

> *While completing my 'A' levels, I have had a part-time job as a waitress at a local restaurant. Through this, I have developed verbal and non-verbal communication skills, learning to deal with customers who on occasions were anxious. I feel these skills will enable me to communicate effectively with the patients I will be responsible for as an adult nurse. I have also learned how to work as part of a team and understand that by collaborating with others, I can achieve better results. Again, these skills will enable me to work as a team with fellow students and colleagues on placement. I have also learned about myself and have developed better time management and prioritising skills, which will help me to complete the theory aspect of studying at university.*

As already identified in Chapter 1, nursing is a very broad term, covering different fields of practice with diversity in each field for example, covering general and specialist areas. In your personal statement, you need to demonstrate that you fully understand the breadth of nursing within your chosen field. Here you can demonstrate your reading and researching into your chosen field of practice. You can also demonstrate your understanding that as a nursing student you will complete community practice learning as well as hospital-based practice learning, and that you really understand the difference between nursing and caring.

Jo Rouse

The personal overtakes the political

This is a tricky one – many prospective candidates are drawn to the professions because of direct experience of being consumers of them. Spending time in hospital with your child as he recovers from having his appendix removed, or supporting your mother as she slides deeper into dementia, will bring you into contact with a vast array of healthcare practitioners. These include nurses, physiotherapists, social carers, theatre practitioners to name but a few, and their professional skills, knowledge and caring can serve as a powerful magnet. You may have thought: 'I could do that'; 'I would like to help people like that'; 'That looks so rewarding'. There is nothing wrong with being inspired like this *but* the application of that inspiration must be handled very carefully on paper. Before we think about that particular task, download the NMC Code from the NMC website (**www.nmc-uk.org**) and refer to it as you consider the following:

What you see from the outside ...	What they see from the inside ...	What the Code says ...
The skills inherent in the nursing care given to your child look smooth and seamless.	The nurse has spent three years learning her/his craft; is supported by a wider multi-disciplinary team; undergoes a programme of continuing professional development.	*40. You must keep your knowledge and skills up to date throughout your working life.*
The nurses caring for your child look happy working within their team and wear a smart uniform.	Nurses have a professional obligation to inspire confidence in the public and to work within a team.	*24. You must work cooperatively within teams and respect the skills, expertise and contributions of your colleagues.*

What you see from the outside ...	What they see from the inside ...	What the Code says ...
The carers supporting your mother are kind, friendly and helpful.	All healthcare practitioners must maintain professional boundaries with the people they care for, because: · Closer relationships with vulnerable people are highly inappropriate; · It is important for them to protect their emotional health; · Being responsible for the care and support of people at the beginning or end of their lives can be very challenging.	*1. You must treat people as individuals and respect their dignity.* *18. You must refuse any gifts, favours or hospitality that might be interpreted as an attempt to gain preferential treatment*
The carers who visit your mother each day at home have their own caseload and are based in the community.	Community-based care can afford practitioners a greater degree of independence and decision making, yet the scope of practice can be challenging.	*38. You must have the knowledge and skills for safe and effective practice when working without direct supervision.*

How then, do you balance your rationale for wanting to become a nurse against your personal experiences or perspectives?

Many admissions tutors would argue that any personal experiences should not be included within the PS because they cloud objectivity or a realistic understanding of the profession itself. For example, what do the following examples tell you about the motivation of the candidates?

I have always wanted to be a midwife since the births of my children. The care I received was fantastic and I think working within the maternity services would be an amazing opportunity to help women go through the most amazing experience of their lives.

Nursing is a beautiful profession and one that I have always admired, especially since watching Holby City.

I became interested in sick children's nursing following the birth of my daughter at 28 weeks' gestation. Louise spent 6 weeks in NICU and during this time, I saw at first hand the importance of the role of the nurse.

Although these are fictional extracts, they are representative of a size-able number of applications received by admissions tutors and will almost always be rejected. The problem with all of these is not that the candidates' motivation is drawn from their own perspective – this can be an excellent starting point – rather that they are unable to elaborate further on how that perspective sits outside a narrow personal box. Essentially, a PS dominated by personal experiences cannot demonstrate an objective motivation:

- Is childbirth really the best experience of all women's lives?
- Does the media portray an accurate picture of nurses?
- How does the care you received from a nurse or midwife translate to the experiences of others?

So, tread very carefully at this stage of the PS. It makes good sense to engage the services of a critical reader with all aspects of your PS and especially at this point. However, it is best not to ask your friends or family who love you and will find it hard or impossible to be objective – your tutor at college, a connexions adviser, or careers officer are much more appropriate people to ask for an opinion.

Of the three examples given above, the final one shows most potential and the first paragraph could be continued as follows:

I became interested in sick children's nursing following the birth of my daughter at 28 weeks' gestation. Louise spent 6 weeks in NICU and during this time, I saw at first hand the importance of the role of the nurse in providing support and comfort to highly anxious parents. During the course of my Access studies, and since obtaining experience as a health-care assistant working within end of life care, I have begun to develop the key nursing skills of care, compassion and communication further. For example...

Note that this candidate has allocated just two short sentences to her/his own personal experiences as a consumer of the health service, and avoided the use of adjectives that imply a value or judgement – *fantastic, amazing, wonderful* for example. The writer then frees her/himself up to start to impress the admissions tutor with knowledge of what the key skills required of a nurse working within this environment are, and crucially, what s/he has done to develop that understanding further. As an introduction to the PS as a whole, it has done its job and opens up clear opportunities for the candidate to elaborate further.

Evidence of key skills

You're doing well so far – you have managed to articulate your understanding of your chosen profession, and have balanced your personal motivation with an objective and realistic perspective of that profession. The next task is to offer some evidence of the key skills that you possess in abundance and how they will be directly beneficial to the career path you have chosen. A common error at this point is for candidates to state several times during the PS that they 'have lots of relevant skills' without actually saying what those skills are, and in what context they been have been developed.

Thorough research at the planning stage of the application should have revealed the key attributes of a nurse or midwife – refresh your memory now by revisiting Chapter 1. It won't be possible to address all of these in a word limited PS and therefore the challenge for you at this stage is to pick out and elaborate on some of the more significant ones, for example interpersonal and caring skills. As a minimum, you should easily be able to identify the importance of study skills, time management and team work for example, based on your own recent experiences at school or college. Even if you have limited, or no actual experience of caring for people in a clinical environment, you should still be able to relate some key skills to one or more aspects of your life experience to date. The following examples demonstrate that skilful writing can illuminate not only what your understanding of the skill is, but also how important that skill is to your chosen profession. Note that it is possible to do this, even if the experience doesn't initially appear to 'match' your profession. As you read the extracts, try to identify the range of key skills addressed within them.

In Year 10 at school, I took part in the 'buddy' scheme, an initiative designed to tackle bullying. Through this role, I appreciated the distress caused to younger pupils who experienced bullying and worked hard to act as a positive role model through my behaviour towards them and other pupils. Supporting my peers in this way, as well as regular meetings with the head teacher, developed my communication and assertiveness skills. I understand that sometimes nurses have to act as advocates for vulnerable patients or relatives, and therefore believe that this experience has been a good introduction to the skills of advocacy and diplomacy.

To help my understanding of caring for women in stressful situations, I volunteered for Women's Aid and helped by organising domestic tasks within a local refuge. Encountering vulnerable, and often depressed, women has reinforced my understanding of the importance of empathy in this type of situation, rather than sympathy. Although I found some of the women's stories to be very shocking, I realised the importance of always respecting the women's experiences and acting in a non-judgemental manner. Relating the importance of positive attitudes to midwifery, I understand that one of the key roles of the midwife is to help women manage their pain during labour. My developing empathetic skills should therefore be helpful to women in making the right choices about pain relief at this frequently stressful time.

Don't cheat!

This is a timely point at which to discuss the importance of making the personal statement *your* work. Of course it is acceptable to receive guidance from your course tutor or careers adviser in planning the PS. However, it is not acceptable to copy and paste text from elsewhere, or recycle material used in a previous PS, or ask someone else to write it for you.

UCAS routinely run every PS through anti-plagiarism (cheating) software, and any detections will be forwarded to the relevant university as well as to you. Earlier in this chapter, you looked at the NMC Code and will recall that perhaps the fundamental principle of the professional guidelines that govern nursing and midwifery practice is to 'be open and honest, act with integrity and uphold the reputation of your profession'. Cheating, therefore, hardly fits within this principle and will not impress an Admissions tutor. It is also heavily frowned upon in the academic world and carries potentially serious penalties, for example being discontinued from a course.

Applicants to nursing and midwifery courses may be tempted to cheat with their personal statements, although I have not yet encountered a PS that has been blatantly copied from another source. The 'worst' case I have dealt with is a midwifery candidate who submitted a PS with 60 per cent of the content being an exact copy of one previously submitted. Given that the first PS did not result in successful shortlisting, you would be correct in thinking that this candidate did nothing to increase her chances of success and was in fact, rejected again.

Anecdotally, it is known that parents (or friends) may write a PS for their child, especially for an oversubscribed course like midwifery or child health nursing. Again, this is an example of false economy. Although there may be success at the shortlisting stage, the candidate is very likely to be 'found out' at selection day. For example, I recall a small number of midwifery candidates who were not able to perform in any of the activities at selection stage, yet had submitted personal statements that confidently and succinctly highlighted their communication and interpersonal skills.

In summary, remember that cheating at any stage of your academic and professional life is:

- dishonest;
- lazy;

- unprofessional;
- counterproductive;
- detectable.

Effective writing

We have already briefly begun to explore some of the keys to effective writing of the PS, for example avoiding text that is too personal or contains inappropriate language. It is easy to underestimate the value of a coherent, well-structured and interesting statement when the emphasis is on 'selling' your motivation and commitment to your chosen profession. If you can locate this motivation within an effective piece of writing overall, that pays attention to detail and takes nothing for granted, then you are well on your way to being shortlisted.

Remember that professional people who expect certain standards and will make a judgement of your understanding of professionalism in writing will be reading your PS. This applies to any written communication you have with Admissions tutors, such as by email. Here are some guidelines and examples:

- Don't use adjectives that imply a value or judgement – you want to be objective, not subjective. Common culprits include 'beautiful', 'amazing' and 'wonderful'. Use 'challenging', 'significant' or 'important' instead.
- Always use appropriate terminology and language, and avoid an informal 'chat' style – imagine that this is a piece of work that you have submitted as part of an assignment. It is still possible to covey enthusiasm and passion for your chosen career when writing in a more formalised style – you just need to choose your words carefully. For example, 'I am very much looking forward to meeting the challenges of the midwifery course' reads better than 'I know the midwifery course will be really hard, but I just can't wait to start'.
- Avoid colloquialisms – practitioners use appropriate and professional terminology. For example, 'I have demonstrated some of the skills required when providing effective support and advice to new mums' is much better when 'mums' is replaced by 'mothers' or 'women'.

- Don't use 'text speak' in your PS or indeed *any* written communication, including email – it is out of context and therefore inappropriate.

- Only include information that is not likely to cause offence or irritation to the staff reading it. For example, the UCAS application form asks for a valid email address and many Admissions tutors value this method of fast communication to resolve a query. If the one you normally use is 'sarahlusciouslips@hotmail.com', ask yourself if this really is the most appropriate one to use when applying for a professional course.

Don't make an Admissions tutor's job any harder than it is already, for example:

- Use correct grammar and punctuation – if in doubt, seek help from your course tutor, or connexions adviser. Space out your PS with paragraphs to make reading easier.

- Abide by the UCAS word count rule. If your PS exceeds the space allowed, it will not appear on the form read by Admissions staff – a sentence that disappears off a form is incomplete and therefore its impact is greatly reduced.

- Complete the UCAS form correctly, for example, make sure your academic qualifications appear in the right place and are all included.

- Make sure your spelling is correct – proofread the finished PS, then ask your course tutor to proofread it. Use the spell check tool in your word-processing software, but remember that some terms associated with your chosen profession may not be spelt as you think. In the UK for example, we write 'fetus' rather than 'foetus'. Careful research at the planning stage of your application will minimise this type of error.

- Include an appropriate and relevant reference. This should not be from a member of your family, or a friend for example. Some universities will request a more suitable reference if your application is otherwise good enough for shortlisting. However, others may not be suitable and this could therefore be a costly error. An appropriate reference is one supplied by your course or school tutor.

Sometimes, an employer's reference can be provided. If in doubt, supply both on your application form.

TOP TIPS

- *Seek objective help writing the personal statement – this is not a sign of weakness.*
- *Ensure your motivation appears balanced and objective – don't rely on personal experience.*
- *Make sure you have a realistic understanding of your chosen profession and the demands of the course – clinical placements will be shift work around the 24-hour clock, including weekends and Bank Holidays.*
- *Identify some relevant key skills – tell us not only that you have them, but provide evidence.*
- *Write the PS in a professional and appropriate way – remember that the person reading it is an experienced, professional practitioner and educator.*
- *Proofread your PS for spelling, punctuation and grammatical errors.*

Selection days – a 'bird's-eye' view

My greeting to candidates at selection days always focuses on their successful journey to that precise point in time. They don't know, for example, that they have managed to obtain a place at a university where the ratio of midwifery places to applicants may be as high as 16:1. So, just to arrive is an achievement. However, this greeting does little to alleviate the nervous expectation of the candidates overall. So this section provides a snapshot that aims to alleviate those nerves a little more, by outlining some of the strategies used by universities in their efforts to secure the best possible candidates. These strategies are then thoroughly explored in the next section by Sarah Holling who has many years of experience in helping prepare candidates for interview.

The aim of any selection day is to select those who show most potential for being caring, compassionate and communicative practitioners, as well as those who are most likely to respond positively to the intense challenges of nursing and midwifery courses, complete them, and take their skills out into practice. In the same way that each university will adopt different entry criteria, selection day strategies will also vary. This can be confusing to candidates and it is understandable that they might question what exactly the best method for selecting those precious people is. Just as with decisions that are made in practice with patients/clients, using the current best evidence available, so universities will work with others to adopt a robust, evidence-based approach to their selection processes. However, in the same way that there can be differences of opinion amongst practitioners in interpreting clinical evidence, so too will there be differences in opinion amongst university Admissions staff interpreting the evidence about the 'best' selection method. Consequently, there is a diverse range of tasks and activities that candidates will undergo and these can include all or some of the following:

- an individual interview;
- a group interview;
- a literacy task;
- a numeracy task;
- practical exercises;
- psychometric tests;
- problem-solving tasks;
- presentations.

A daunting range to be sure, and hard to prepare for if you're fortunate enough to secure an invitation to selection days at five different universities. However, do remember that universities adopt different teaching and learning strategies in order to maximise the quality of the student experience, and therefore it is most appropriate to mimic some of those strategies right from the beginning. As an example, some universities base their nursing or midwifery curricula on a strategy known as 'enquiry-based learning', a method that places responsibility on students for developing their learning, rather than being passive consumers of it. For some applicants, such strategies may be the key reason for seeking admission to a particular university and therefore the relevant selection day strategy is actually a taste of what's to come.

A further challenge for a midwifery or nursing admissions process is to balance the screening of candidates for their academic *and* clinical potential – the two don't always match up. This means that the selection day is looking for a range of skills, knowledge and attributes that span the sometimes precarious bridge between theory and practice. We want students who can manage the academic rigours of an undergraduate degree programme, but must also display their abilities to care for people, support them, and be kind to them. Often, the challenges faced by a selection day team are centred on this mismatch of skills range. Some candidates may be accurate with numeracy and literacy, able to obtain full marks and write proficiently, yet be unable to display empathy, or communicate fluently with others. I hope that this book so far has illustrated clearly why such a candidate wouldn't be accepted onto a nursing or midwifery programme.

As part of the invitation letter sent to you, the university should outline the broad structure of the selection day itself – it will certainly direct you with any preparation that you are required to do as part of the activities. Some universities will also send you a comprehensive list of suggested resources to access in advance of the day. Take every opportunity to look at such resources as they will offer big clues about what you will be expected to do. Above all else, don't underestimate the range of skills that will be tested on the day, so ensure that you practise as much as possible. Don't do all this in isolation – speak to your school or college tutors, access their careers advisory service, or visit the extremely helpful staff at *connexions*. Although these people may not have a full understanding of the profession you're seeking to enter they will have lots of useful tips and advice to share with you, based on their years of experience at supporting students going through university interviews.

Earlier in the chapter, I outlined some general advice about completing the personal statement, and this should have given you an overview of what a selection day team will be 'testing' on the day. As a minimum, this will be your motivation to become a student nurse or midwife and your understanding of the profession itself. The ways in which universities 'test' their candidates will vary, as discussed earlier. However, you can be sure that just like the personal statement, the motivation must be objective, and the understanding broad. At Worcester, we ask candidates to prepare an item that represents their motivation to become a midwife, and be ready to share it with the other candidates on the day. The candidates who do best at this are those who have:

- adhered to the advice to prepare in advance;
- sought advice and support from others;
- ensured that their item was suitable for sharing (some have been questionable);
- been objective;
- related the item clearly to their personal motivation to enter the profession.

Of course, we fully appreciate that this can be a tough task to do under 'interview' conditions – they can be very stressful days and candidates often put themselves under tremendous pressure to succeed. However, a well-organised candidate who has a very clear picture of the type of midwife they want to be because they've done their homework, will actually find this task a relative breeze. After all, haven't you been spending most of your recent life telling everyone how much you want to be a nurse or midwife, and why you're going to be good at it?

So, what skills, knowledge and attributes are a selection day team looking for? You may not believe this, but selection day teams are actually human – they *want* you to succeed, and will of course make allowances for nerves and look hard for evidence of potential. Remember that they are also very experienced nurses and midwives, as well as being educators, and are thus ideally placed to make an assessment of candidate performance. However, we don't presume to get it right all the time and don't make decisions about people's futures in isolation. As it is good practice, a variety of other stakeholders are usually involved in the selection process and these include educators, clinicians, students and healthcare consumers. Essentially, people who fully understand the full range of skills expected of students in the dual worlds of theory and practice.

This multi-disciplinary approach provides an opportunity for you, the nursing or midwifery candidate, to showcase the full range of talents that you possess, or will possess with careful nurturing once you're on the course. Midwifery candidates at Worcester are provided with a 'job description' (see Box 3.2) that offers some significant clues about what key characteristics the selection day team are looking for.

Box 3.2 Selection day 'job description' of key characteristics required of midwifery candidate at Worcester

1. Interpersonal skills:
   - oral communication;
   - empathy;
   - kindness;
   - reflective;
   - considerate;
   - confident;
   - responsive.
2. Professionalism:
   - professional appearance;
   - honesty/integrity;
   - emotional maturity;
   - self-confidence;
   - respect;
   - organisational skills.
3. Motivational fit:
   - realistic understanding of role;
   - positive attitude;
   - enthusiasm;
   - cheerful;
   - flexible;
   - stamina.

4. Problem-solving skills:
  - initiative;
  - tact and diplomacy;
  - negotiation and persuasion;
  - collaborative;
  - assertiveness.
5. Skills and ability:
  - numerical ability;
  - written communication;
  - personal insight/self-awareness.

This 'job description' could equally apply to nursing candidates and if you revisit the student nurses' opinions in Chapter 1, you will indeed observe several matches. If you are provided with a person specification like this one, do please read it carefully, think about it, and act upon it. For example, if you are not confident at speaking up in front of strangers, or the thought of doing it makes you feel quite ill, move yourself immediately out of your comfort zone and *practise*. One of the best ways to do this is by volunteering to help someone out, whether this is your local Brownies group, or in a residential home, or through one of the excellent peer development opportunities that are becoming more widely available within schools. Remember that a specification such as this will form the basis of the assessment tools used by the selection day team, as well as give you some hefty clues about what will be expected of you on the day. However, a word to the wise – some of these attributes could be developed as part of the process of becoming a midwife or nurse; others must be fundamental to your essential self. By this stage of the book, you should easily be able to work out the latter.

Rejection

Sometimes, despite your best efforts, the decision made by the selection day team is 'no'. Everybody, at some stage of their lives, is not successful at what they're trying to achieve at the first attempt. Although this is extremely disappointing, the trick is not to run away and lie down in a dark room, but learn from the experience and move on. In Chapter 4, we look at the concept of emotional intelligence (EI) and your reaction to a 'no' is a good test of your EI. Like most admissions tutors, I have seen a range of responses from people who haven't received the news they wanted or expected. In my experience, this can take shape as:

- A highly emotional reaction – crying, pleading with staff for another chance etc.
- Blaming someone else for the rejection – complaining that the process wasn't fair, someone else was treated differently etc.
- Reflecting on the feedback provided, asking for direction about how to improve, and looking forward to another chance.

The first two are understandable responses to disappointment and frustration, especially when the stakes are high – essentially 'knee jerk' responses. What you're aiming for is the third option, and I do see far more of this one than the other two. In my experience, most universities will provide feedback about your overall performance at selection day. It may have been, for example, that you were unable to showcase your skills effectively because you were overwhelmingly nervous; or, the communication exercise that you took part in demonstrated that your interpersonal skills are not yet developed enough to withstand the demands of caring for patients/clients. Any feedback you receive should outline issues such as these and therefore act as a springboard for you to:

- reflect on the day's activities;
- be honest about how well you think you did;
- think about how to refine the areas that you didn't perform as well in;
- seek help in making them better;
- practise them;
- then try again next year.

Of course, it may be that the feedback indicates that your skills, knowledge and attributes do not match those required of a nurse or midwifery student. Reflect on it carefully. This is where the service of your critical reader can be employed again, as it is hard for us to be truly self-critical; the human race is very good at fooling itself. If, for example, your feedback indicates that empathy or caring behaviour was not demonstrated as part of the selection day tasks, then you should think about a different career pathway. These particular skills, crucial to the role of a nurse and midwife, really cannot be taught.

How to be successful at interview

Sarah Holling

Candidates often assume that getting an offer is *only* about doing well at the selection stage; it isn't. The interview is important but often you need to perform well in a range of different tests. No one will expect you to be perfect, but you need to be confident attempting each of the activities you may be asked to do.

Pre-interview 'basics'

On receiving an interview offer, you should immediately confirm attendance. You may be turned away from your interview if the university has no record that you have confirmed your attendance, or if you confirm too late. So, if you haven't done so, accept the invitation now. You can always cancel at a later date if necessary.

Be polite when calling; you could be talking to someone who will make a decision about your application. Note down their name. Never rely on leaving a phone message or a phone call; always send an email or write a letter to provide a written confirmation. Make sure emails and letters are error free. Include: your full name; course title and UCAS code if possible; interview date; your address; contact telephone number; UCAS application number. Keep a record of all conversations, times and dates, and copies of emails and letters. Put these in your file. Written proof is invaluable in resolving problems.

If you have a **disability**, when you accept your invitation remind Admissions. If you are dyslexic or dyspraxic you may be offered extra time to complete tests, or the use of a dictionary.

You will normally need to take **original documents** (plus often photocopies) of documents with you. What is required will vary. It is very important you do *exactly* what is required; if the instructions say bring *two* photocopies of each original then do so!

If you have problems locating originals you *must* contact the university well in advance. If you cannot find exam certificates, obtaining a replacement from an exam board can take months. If you have to reapply for any documents make sure you keep a record of all phone calls, emails and letters so that you provide these as proof to the university. Arriving with everything as instructed demonstrates your organisational skills.

If you are completing your **Criminal Records Bureau (CRB)** form at the interview, taking your documents with you is particularly important. If your course requires that you will go out into practice early in your first term, a delay in obtaining CRB clearance could cause serious problems. So, make a list of what documents you will need. Check which you have and tick them off on the Interview Checklist provided on pages 98–99. An A4 plastic popper file is great for keeping all these documents safe and in one place.

Doing your research

Research doesn't end when you submit your personal statement. Being well informed gives you an advantage over other candidates and helps you make the right course choice. You need to think again now about your chosen profession and the courses for which you have applied. To help you with this task, now work through Activity 3.1.

ACTIVITY 3.1

Reviewing your application

Reread your personal statement. Why do you want to do the course? Has anything changed? For example, you may now have some new voluntary experience. What haven't you explained adequately?

What questions do you still have? What worries do you have?

Note these down; some may be questions you ask at interview.

Suggested selection day resources can be found on page 100. Always consider how current and relevant information is. Make sure you have looked carefully at the university's website. Be selective about the Internet and the type of questions you read or post on discussion boards.

You are likely to be asked to discuss current issues in your profession either at interview, or to write about them in your literacy test. More advice on this follows later. Be aware of what is in the news. Know about key Department of Health reports and proposed changes. Look again at the suggested reading provided in this book, and don't forget your historical timeline in Chapter 1. Activity 3.2 will help you to prepare.

ACTIVITY 3.2

Researching current issues

Look at some nursing/midwifery journals. Read a local paper and/or look at the Internet. Identify several topical issues. Make notes and form an opinion. Be able to discuss the different aspects or viewpoints. Make sure they are relevant.

This demonstrates important skills, including: commitment to evidence-based practice; appreciation of equality; motivation; ability to research; critical thinking and verbal communication. Be prepared to explain why you picked these topics.

You may be asked why you selected a particular course or university. Researching allows you to make the right choice. It also shows the interviewer 'buying intent', that is, how genuinely interested you are. Now do Activity 3.3.

ACTIVITY 3.3

Reviewing your course/university choice

What do you know about the course or university? What do you think is likely to be important? Who else's views should you consider? Review your open day checklist from Chapter 2.

Now look again at your checklist and put an 'E' next to things that are very important/essential. Are there other things that are 'nice to have'/ preferable? Put a 'P' next to them. Keep your list safe as you will keep returning to this.

If you have not yet attended an open day then try to do so. Some interviews will include a campus tour; find out if this is included.

Travel to selection day

An important part of preparing for selection day is working out how to get there, and how to be on time. To help with your planning and preparation:

- obtain timetables (helpful if your bus or train is cancelled on the day);
- find out the cost of the fare. How will you pay?
- obtain a campus map;
- investigate car parking (if relevant) – how much does it cost?
- find out exactly where the interview is on campus;
- make a back-up plan in case of strikes or travel disruption;
- calculate your journey time – and add an extra 50 per cent on to this;
- always plan to arrive at least 30 minutes before the time instructed.

If possible, do a dry run to check your travel plans, and where you are going on campus. This will give you a lot of confidence on the day. You may not want your family to go with you, but this may make travelling easier. However, plan what they will do while you are at your interview as they will not be able to accompany you.

Whatever you do – **do not be late**. Punctuality is a very important professional skill and being late will reflect badly on you. The admissions team may even turn you away on the day. However, if something does go wrong and you are unavoidably delayed, make sure you call the university to let them know and then accept their decision.

Make sure that you **stay safe**. Have loose change and emergency money so that if your travel plans change you have the ability to get safely to the university or home. Make sure someone knows where you are going, and when you should be back. Keep to main roads, and don't be tempted to take short cuts, especially late at night. Never be tempted to dip into your emergency money – unless it is a *real* emergency.

Interview survival kit

You will probably spend a lot of time thinking about what you are going to wear, and hopefully how you will get to your interview. However, there are lots of things you should consider taking with you. Candidates may find it helpful to develop their own 'survival kit' which they take to each interview. So, make a list of items that you think it will be useful to take to interview. Compare your list with the things suggested on page 101. Make sure you have a suitable bag to put these into and start gathering the things you want well before the interview day.

The night before

Hopefully by this stage you are feeling well prepared. Go through your interview checklist, research notes on key topics, reread your interview invitation letter, and if you haven't already done so, pack your bag. Ensure that you have your clothes and shoes ready to wear. Take a little time to review the notes you made at open days about the things you want to find out, and that are important to you about the course you have chosen to do. If you haven't already done so, make sure you have three or four questions you can ask the interviewer.

A good night's sleep is important. Set your alarm clock (and preferably a back up). But if you can't sleep, then accept you are nervous and just get up early. Relax; remind yourself that you have done your preparation and there is no reason for you not to be successful.

Mastering selection tests

All candidates applying for healthcare courses will usually be interviewed, but many will do other activities including:

- maths/numeracy test;
- English/literacy test;
- group exercise;

- personality questionnaire;
- individual presentation;
- question and answer sessions.

The first three items in the above list are the most common activities and are discussed here, although each university will utilise different strategies, as outlined at the beginning of the chapter. However, rapid changes are taking place. Some universities are starting to use personality questionnaires, and a national personality profiling tool is under development in England.

You may ask, 'Why am I being assessed?' Tests give you more chance to prove your suitability for a course. They measure skills that are difficult to assess at interview and/or provide a way for the university to assess a skill in several ways. This makes the outcome fairer; if you suffer from nerves in the interview, you can still demonstrate your excellent communication skills in a group exercise. It also means that everything doesn't rest solely on the outcome of the interview.

Or, perhaps you don't like doing tests. All healthcare professionals undergo continual assessments during training and throughout their career. You need to accept that this is part of the job. If you suffer from severe anxiety, speak to your GP. In most cases, confidence can be improved by practice, and by having a clear understanding of what is being assessed.

TOP TIPS

Questions to ask:

- *Request sample questions/a practice paper if available.*
- *Ask what maths topics are recommended for revision.*
- *Find out about the types of question, such as calculations, interpreting and extracting data from tables, applied questions such as 'how long will it take to get from A to B'?*
- *Is a calculator allowed?*
- *Is there a pass mark?*

During the test:

- *Turn off your mobile phone.*

- *If possible, go to the toilet before starting your test.*

- *Don't be tempted to cheat or copy your neighbour's work.*

- *Follow the instructions on the test paper – make sure there are no questions on the back!*

- *Plan your time. If you have 20 minutes and 20 questions you should have done half of the questions in the first 10 minutes.*

- *Don't assume that the questions get harder; if you can't do a question then move quickly on to the next question.*

- *If you do not answer or miss a question be very careful that your subsequent answers are next to the correct question number.*

- *Circle any questions you are not sure about with a pencil. This will help you locate them quickly if you have time later to have another attempt.*

- *If you are not clear on the instructions – ask the administrator.*

- *Make sure you have spare pens and pencils.*

- *Have a watch – you may not be able to see the clock in the room.*

- *Clearly show your 'working out' in maths questions, or your plan if writing an essay if instructed.*

- *Will you be penalised for wrong answers? If not it is always worth taking a guess at answers.*

- *Check you have converted to the correct unit of measurement. If you are asked to give the answer in grams do not give it in milligrams.*

- *Do a rough check of your answers if time allows. In numeracy tests this is particular important. For example: if you are asked to calculate 76 + 23, round 76 to 80, then round 23 to 20. The answer will be around 100. If your answer is much higher or lower it should tell you that it is probably wrong. This is quicker than actually redoing the maths for each question.*

Maths/numeracy tests

Increasing emphasis is placed on basic numeracy and testing of this vital skill at selection, and is indeed a requirement demanded by the NMC. Nurses and midwives perform specific types of drug calculations as part of their daily practice. When a patient's life is involved, 100 per cent accuracy is vital. For this reason most universities use numeracy tests.

Links to sample tests and revision tools are provided in the resources section on page 100. Candidates must know what skills are required, and what topics are covered. Some universities provide a lot of guidance including a practice paper.

If you are one of the people who say 'I wasn't good at maths at school', fortunately the skills needed for healthcare are very specific – you only need to master certain topics. Many excellent free resources are on the Internet for improving numeracy. If this area is a weakness, do some numeracy assessment tests and get advice. Try speaking to a careers adviser, teacher, the admissions tutor, or LearnDirect for help. Universities now offer much help but you need to know how to take advantage of it.

Some maths skills you may need to revise include the following:

- terminology – e.g. improper fraction, decimal, factor, simplify, cancel, convert;
- basic arithmetic skills – addition, subtraction, multiplication and long division;
- sequence of operations (BoDMAS);
- converting fractions to decimals (and vice versa);
- multiplying, adding, subtracting simple fractions;
- cancelling and simplifying fractions;
- rounding and decimal places;
- units of measurement, e.g. grams, kilograms, litres and millilitres and converting between them.

Box 3.3 Example maths/numeracy questions

- 876/12
- 13.6 + 87.5
- John is prescribed an antibiotic. He has to take 500 mg once a day for 7 days. How many grams of antibiotic will he have taken at the end of 7 days?
- Convert 3/5 to a percentage.

English/literacy tests

These tend to take one of four different forms and you may encounter several in one paper. The four question types are the following:

- Correcting spelling/grammar mistakes in a paragraph.
- Filling in the 'right word'. For example, 'Do you have any experience of/on/for giving injections?'
- Comprehension – questions based on a paragraph of text.
- Essay (the topic may be given to you in advance, or on the day). There is normally only one topic but it is phrased so that most candidates will be able to write something.

The essay seems to cause the most concern to candidates. It is not just about writing something engaging. Originality and good research (if you are given the topic in advance) will only get you so far. Other things that are assessed are:

- grammatical or spelling errors;
- keeping to the word count;
- completing the essay in the time provided;
- having a clear structure;
- legibility of handwriting;
- following instructions;

- maintaining a balance between personal experience and objective discussion;
- understanding of the profession and the skills required;
- need for non-discriminatory practice.

Try to incorporate references to key documents such as the NMC Code into your essay to demonstrate you have taken the time to look at this. Use your time carefully, dividing it to include: reading the question, planning an answer (use bullet points or a mind map), writing the answer, and checking your writing. Allocate two-thirds of your time to writing. Never cross out your plan until you are sure you have finished; if you run out of time it will show what you would have written. Ensure that your *essay* is clearly differentiated from your *plan* to avoid confusion.

Group exercises

Group exercises can take many forms including:

- A practical task – usually with a time limit – such as building something from plastic blocks following a diagram.
- A discussion where you will be asked to consider a problem or topic.
- A 'who/what would you take with you' exercise – for example, if trapped on a desert island, or going to live on the moon!

A common mistake is to be overly focused on the outcome – the interviewer is more interested in how you work in a team, and what you do, than the end result; multi-disciplinary and team working are very important in healthcare.

Thinking about the skills that are being assessed in group exercises can help candidates perform well. These may include:

- how you share out/allocate tasks;
- working under pressure and managing time;
- awareness of current issues in healthcare and the standards expected;
- verbal communication skills;
- ability to listen to others;
- respecting the views of others/empathy;

- supporting others and encouraging them;
- problem-solving skills – ability to generate ideas;
- sense of humour;
- determination.

Important things to consider in group exercises include the following:

- Speak clearly and slowly. Maintain eye contact with the group. Be prepared to discuss your ideas, and be able to back them up.
- Do not get into disputes. If there is a disagreement, present both options to the group and take a vote. Accept the decision and work positively towards achieving the outcome.
- Working to deadlines is important. You might want to volunteer to keep an eye on time, or suggest how you will organise your time.
- Allow others the opportunity to talk. If you find that one or two people dominate the discussion try to move the conversation on. For example, you could summarise what they have said and then ask someone else for their opinion.
- While your contribution is important – you must be prepared to say or do something – equally important is how you encourage others to be involved and respect their views. Ensure you are listening to what everyone has to say. Do not eat sweets, chew gum, use your phone during this or any other activity, or doodle on a pad.
- You may want to try to summarise the discussion at the end of the exercise, or take the lead in deciding how to tackle a task.
- Don't be disheartened if you weren't the 'leader' for the task. Healthcare is about working together and not everyone can be in charge. You will not be penalised. In fact, candidates who 'over dominate' group tasks to the detriment of the rest of the group are often marked down.

Mastering an interview

Treat every interview like your first

The good news is that if you have got an interview the university wants to recruit you! The personal statement has done its job; but, there may be anywhere between three and ten candidates chasing each place. So, how can you make yourself memorable and get the offer? Whether this is your first interview, or if you consider yourself an 'old hand' you must prepare for each interview separately, because each course is different.

It will come as no surprise by now that the secret is in good preparation. Interviewing is like riding a bike. It's a skill. It takes time to develop, and you can get a bit wobbly unless you practise! But practice makes perfect. Your school or college should be able to offer help. Always take this. Alternatively, a friend or relative may have some experience of doing interviews. Now do Activity 3.4 to help with your interview preparation.

ACTIVITY 3.4

Interview preparation recap

Do you know the key details about your interview? Specifically:

- duration of the interview?
- number of interviewer/s?
- name/job role of interviewer/s?
- where/when the interview will be held?

Dress for success

Buying a suit can be expensive and you are not expected to wear one. However, if you do buy one, choose something neutral, such as a dark colour that will not mark easily. Here are some other tips for appropriate dressing for the interview.

If in doubt, dress 'up' rather than 'down'. A suit can easily be made less formal by removing a jacket. Looking good will make you feel confident. Steer away from anything that is too trendy. You need to look tidy and professional. Jeans, T-shirts and shorts are definitely inappropriate, as are flip-flops and trainers.

Your clothes and shoes must be comfortable. If any of these are too tight you will not have a pleasant day. You could be doing a lot of walking on the day, so shoes need to be practical rather than high fashion. Take a lightweight jacket that is easy to carry around all day.

Regarding personal hygiene and jewellery, a safe maxim is to apply the same standards that would be required by a student on placement. Keep jewellery to a minimum (maximum one set of stud earrings, no necklaces) and make sure you wear a reliable deodorant if you use one because you will probably perspire more under pressure! Your clothes should be clean and ironed. Shoes should be polished. Remove all rings except a wedding ring. Get a haircut and make sure any facial hair is smart. Healthcare is one of the few courses where a professional appearance is likely to be assessed at interview.

Interview stages and interviewers

Interviews have three clear stages: the beginning, middle and end.

At the beginning, the interviewer will welcome you and introduce the people who are present. They may ask if you have anything that needs to be sorted out before you start. For example, you may need to go to the toilet (it is much better to deal with this before you go into the interview, but it happens!). The interviewers should explain to you how long the interview will last and when you can ask questions. Convention dictates you should leave any questions until the end.

The middle part of the interview is where *you* will answer questions. Usually the panel will start with one or two 'easy' questions to help you relax.

At the end, this is where you may be given the opportunity to ask questions (see Activity 3.5). The interviewers should explain when you will find out the result. If not, you can ask them. This is also a good time to thank them for the opportunity to interview, and reiterate that you would accept any offer and that you are still very interested.

ACTIVITY 3.5

Questions to ask at interview

If you haven't already done so, make a list of the things you would like to ask at interview. You should have no more than three or four questions.

Candidates are often worried about what to do if there is more than one interviewer, called a panel interview. Interviewers may be teaching staff, clinicians, students and healthcare users. One of the interviewers will usually be the chair and will 'lead' the interview. Address the person who asks each question. At the end of the question then make eye contact with the other panel members. Each person will usually have specific questions they will ask.

Interview etiquette

Just like learning to drive, or sitting an exam, there are certain interview conventions:

- Do not be late! Arrive 15 minutes before your allotted time slot.
- Shaking hands. A firm handshake while making eye contact is important. Do not shake the interviewer's hand so hard they are left with bruised fingers!
- Do not sit down until instructed. You should check if necessary where they want you to sit – don't move the chair.
- Avoid creating distractions. Do not chew gum, fiddle with jewellery, 'click' a pen, or any other irritating and distracting tic.
- Switch off your phone. Never answer it during an interview. If there is a real emergency and you are expecting a call such as due to a sick child, then explain the situation to the interviewer.
- Don't get into an argument. If the interviewer makes an incorrect statement about you then politely correct them. They may say that you got a grade E in Biology when in fact you got a B. It is appropriate to correct this. The interviewer may have just misread the application. Offer your certificate for checking or to send them corroborating documentation after the interview.
- Maintain eye contact – but don't 'stare'. And even if you are disinterested in the interview, do not allow this to show. They have invested time and money in pursuing your application.
- Do not criticise colleagues or blame others for problems. Take responsibility for what has happened. Demonstrate that you have learnt from mistakes and what you would do/have done differently. We all make mistakes; it is how we learn from them that counts.
- Never use bad language or jargon. It is poor practice to use medical jargon with patients as it can be a block to understanding; similarly avoid it in interview. It can also come across as pretentious.

- Avoid boasting about achievements. If the interviewer congratulates you about something, a simple 'thank you' and a smile is sufficient. Never try to appear more qualified than your interviewer.

- Don't talk too much! Some candidates ruin their chances by talking for too long, either because of overenthusiasm, nerves or a need to impress. They fail to pick up on body language from the interviewer which is then followed by verbal cues. These may include: 'this is very interesting but we do need to move onto other areas'; or 'unfortunately we have only a limited amount of time today. Can we now discuss ...'. This marks the applicant down because they lack interpersonal awareness.

- Do not interrupt the interviewer.

- Watch your body language. Do not fold your arms, fiddle with your fingers or hair. There are many good books written on body language, but do not become too obsessed with this as it may increase your anxiety!

- Avoid becoming emotional. Healthcare professionals must be able to separate personal emotions from professional situations. An interview is not a counselling session.

- Leave mum at home! Some parents do want to go to the interview so that they can see the campus and facilities. Arrange somewhere to meet them afterwards.

- Do not be over-familiar. Address all staff by their title – e.g. Mr, Mrs or Dr – and be careful about using first names, even if the interviewer uses their first name or addresses a colleague by their first name.

- **Never lie**. Sadly a few candidates try to hide things that would exclude them. They are almost always found out and risk being forced to leave the course. A student could be found unfit to practise at the end of three years due to something that is discovered as late as their third year. It is also a **criminal offence** to make a false application. Be honest about health problems, criminal convictions or cautions, exams taken and exam results, or previous attempts at doing the course elsewhere.

What sort of questions will be asked?

A good range of possible interview questions are provided at the end of the chapter on page 102.

You have very little time. In a 30-minute interview you will probably answer no more than five or six questions. Make what you say **count**. The interviewer has many candidates to see. Keep to the point and help them to do their job.

An example question is 'Why do you want to do become a midwife?' This question gives you the opportunity to demonstrate:

- how you have researched the career;
- that you understand midwifery focuses on the care of a woman and her family;
- examples of how you have the key aptitudes needed;
- work experience or insight experiences/visits you have made;
- your motivation and enthusiasm

Dealing with tricky moments

Every interview will throw up at least one question you didn't expect. Don't let this panic you, but practise how you will deal with this. Here are some examples:

- Didn't hear what was asked? Say: 'Sorry, I didn't quite catch that – could you please repeat the question?'
- Don't understand the question? Ask the interviewer to clarify what they want.
- Not sure what to say? Ask them if you could just have a moment to think.
- Still struggling for an answer? Explain you are nervous. Could they perhaps give you a little more guidance? Often the interviewer will say something to get you started on the right path to the answer.
- **You really don't have a clue?** Apologise. Say it is something that you haven't looked into, or not previously considered and that you will look into it further after the interview. Don't despair if this happens. The interviewer will be impressed if you keep calm. You can even turn this into a positive by emailing Admissions after the

GET INTO NURSING AND MIDWIFERY

interview and following up on the question by showing you have gone away and looked into it.

When things have gone wrong

Candidates often make the mistake of trying to cover up when things have gone wrong such as poor grades, dropping out of a course, or a criminal conviction. But in fact you have a great opportunity to turn this to your advantage.

For example: you got a grade E at GCSE Maths. You know that numeracy is an important skill. Compare these two answers:

Candidate A: Yes I got a grade E – but that's not actually a fail. I'm sure I'll be ok on the course though.

Candidate B: I got a grade E – I did well in all my other exams, but I really struggled with maths. I enrolled on a distance learning course last year, and have just resat it. I am predicted a B.

Candidate A tells the interviewer nothing they don't already know, and offers a weak assurance they will do better. Candidate B shows that they have learnt from this, have taken the initiative to do something about their grade, and that they are likely to achieve the grade needed. It also updates the interviewer about information they may not have. Candidate B is more likely to receive an offer, conditional on their result.

How can you improve your chances of getting an offer?

For popular courses you really need to stand out to the interviewer. Firstly you need to 'tick all the boxes' – professional appearance, be punctual, bring what was asked, and understand interview etiquette.

If you really take time to think through the skills needed in the profession, and all the different experience you have gained, you are likely to do well. For popular courses you *must* know about the course, the placement hospitals and their strengths, and what you can bring to the course. Reflect on your life experience, visits, journal articles you have read; these can all give your interview something unique. You must tailor your answers to each course/interview, and make sure you are actually talking about the right university/course if you are going to several interviews close together!

If possible mention something new at interview that you haven't included in your UCAS application, such as work experience you have now gained. It will get the attention of the interviewer who may be on their eighth interview of the day!

Finally always have a written list of questions to ask the interviewer. These should be about things you cannot read about in the prospectus or website (refer back to the list you made in Activity 3.5).

TOP TIPS

- *If asked, tell the interviewer about other offers. However, be clear that if you get an offer this is the course you want to do. Otherwise, the interviewer may feel that there is no point making you an offer.*

- *Stop and ask yourself is this the 'right place' for you? Don't be taken in by glossy brochures and facilities. Go back to your list of 'essentials' and make sure that the course fulfils all of these. Remember, the interview is a two-way process.*

- *You will get out what you put in. If you work through the activities in this chapter and make sure you are fully prepared you should stand a good chance of securing at least one offer.*

- *The university wants you. The interview just helps confirm they are making the right decision. Be yourself - enjoy the day!*

Post-interview tasks

On your way home or when you get home, you will be tired but there is *still* some work to do!

First impressions

These are often forgotten within hours of leaving the university. So, as soon as you are able to, complete Activity 3.6.

ACTIVITY 3.6

First impressions

Write down your first impressions and memories of the following:

- What went well?
- What went wrong?
- Names of people you met?
- Information you didn't previously know.
- What interview questions did you get asked?
- What did you have to do for the tests?
- What did you like?
- What worries do you have?
- Would you accept an offer?
- When will you know the outcome?
- Things you didn't know or have changed?

It's important to be critical. If the university was disorganised or is slow to make a decision about your application, does this mean that the course will also be badly organised?

What has the university asked you to do?

You may have been told to do various things, such as provide copies of results or certificates. Make sure you do this straight away and always send information with a letter or by email so you have proof. If you are posting something it must go 'Signed For'. If you have been told that you may be placed on a waiting list make sure you write to say you are still interested. Check they have your contact details in Admissions, and follow up regularly with them. Every year people get their chosen course after being on a waiting list but it requires determination.

Rate your courses/universities

Now is the time to rank your applications. As you go to each interview put them in order. Which one is your first choice, which is your second? If you do this as you go along, it will be much easier to make a decision if you are lucky enough to get more than one offer.

So all that now remains is for you to sit back and wait for your offer ... and good luck!

'I'm worried that I won't get a place because I have dyslexia/a criminal conviction/a health problem'

Not every application received by Admissions tutors is straight-forward – some are from applicants who are anxious because they have had a previous criminal conviction, others because they have a disability such as dyslexia. This doesn't automatically rule you out from obtaining a place on a nursing or midwifery course, but it does require an open and honest approach from both the university and you. The NMC issue guidance to help support Admissions tutors when assessing candidates with these types of issues and any deci-sion made is not done in isolation. This guidance is known as the *Good Health and Good Character* document and can be accessed via the NMC's website (www.nmc-uk.org).

Remember that the law for people with disabilities is on your side. The Equality Act of 2010 makes it illegal for employers in business, the public and private sectors (that includes universities) to discrimi-nate against a person because of a disability, and operates under the concept of *reasonable adjustments*. Put simply, this means that employ-ers cannot presume that an employee cannot safely and effectively perform their job by virtue of having a disability. The guiding principle should be: can the person fulfil the requirements of their job if rea-sonable adjustments have been made? Examples of what these might be are discussed below. You can read more about the Equality Act at http://www.equalities.gov.uk/Default.aspx

All successful candidates to a nursing or midwifery programme have to undergo an enhanced criminal records bureau (CRB) check, and this will identify *any* incident that involved a caution or conviction, even if it occurred some years ago and the person has subsequently been 'clean' and the conviction spent. It is therefore best to be upfront about any caution/conviction you have received from the outset, and the UCAS application form invites you to do just that. Declaring a caution or conviction does not automatically mean that your application will be rejected. Remember that one of the questions guiding Admissions tutors is 'Has the candidate disclosed the caution or conviction?', therefore honesty really is the best policy.

To help illuminate how these processes work, here are some fictional case studies, loosely based on the experiences of real applicants.

Would you offer these candidates a place on your course?

Criminal conviction/caution

Gary

Gary is 26 years old and applying for a place on a mental health nursing programme.

At the age of 14, Gary was caught shoplifting and received a police caution. He has not received any further cautions or convictions since. He has declared this incident to the Admissions tutor, expressing his anxiety that it won't 'count against him'.

Case study 3.1

Using the guidance established by the NMC guidelines (see **http://www .nmc-uk.org/Educators/Good-health-and-good-character/**) we can see that the risk posed to patients/service users would be deemed as low, and this incident is highly unlikely to prevent Gary from obtaining a place on the mental health nursing programme, if he goes on to be successful at selection.

The key issues informing this decision would be based on the following:

● Gary has not repeated the offence and therefore a pattern of offending has not been established.
● 12 years have elapsed since the shoplifting occurred.
● Gary has declared the caution.

Laura

Laura is 32 and recently applied for a place on a midwifery under-graduate degree programme. At the age of 30, Laura was found guilty of claiming goods under a false name, and ordered to pay a substantial fine, as well as costs. A similar episode occurred four years previously. Laura declared her convictions at the applica-tion stage.

This is not so straightforward. Even though Laura has declared her convictions, note the relatively short amount of time that has elapsed since; her age when they occurred, the pattern of offending, and the nature of the offences themselves. Remember that as a registered mid-wife, you must 'be open and honest, act with integrity and uphold the reputation of your profession'.

Although student midwives are not accountable for their practice until they qualify, the general principles of the NMC Code will still be applied to students, as honesty and trustworthiness are required from the very begin-ning of a professional career. Laura is therefore not likely to obtain a place at this time, although she may not necessarily be excluded permanently.

Disability

Jo

Jo is 19 and has dyslexia. She is attending an interview to be a child health nurse, and has declared her dyslexia to the university Admissions team before her attendance at the interview. Part of the interview process involves a literacy task.

Being upfront about her dyslexia means that Jo will be entitled to additional time when completing the literacy task. The Admissions team must then ask themselves two extremely important questions during their initial assessment of Jo:

- Is accurate writing an essential part of the role of a child health nurse?
- Can reasonable adjustments be made so that a child health nurse with dyslexia can be supported to be safe and competent in practice?

The answers to these questions are 'definitely' and 'probably'. Being able to record contemporaneous notes is a statutory requirement of nurses and midwives and is therefore a key skill. Jo's ability to manage her dyslexia will determine the level of support that she will require in practice, for example a mentor proofreading her notes, or practising frequently used terminology. This is not an insurmountable issue but does require careful planning, as the process of organising reasonable adjustments can only be done properly through a multi-disciplinary approach. The NMC are clear in their guidance that the imperative is to balance the safety of the public alongside sound anti-discriminatory policies/practices.

John

John is 42 and applying to join an adult nurse graduate diploma programme. For much of his adult life, John has experienced bouts of depressive illness, and is concerned that if he declares this, he will not be successful in obtaining a place on the programme.

Case study 3.4

It is unsurprising that John is anxious about disclosing his mental illness. Even though many of us will experience some kind of mental illness at some point in our lives, negative and stereotyped attitudes persist.

Essentially, the same principles applied to Jo's application can be applied here – an individualised approach, sensitive to the safety of the public and anti-discriminatory:

- What strategies does John have in place for managing his depression?
- Can he be supported in practice during times of illness?
- Who else needs to be involved?

Like Jo managing her dyslexia, John will understand and manage his depression better than anyone else – it is therefore highly inappropriate (and against the law) to deny him a place unless the decision is based on sound evidence that he would be unable to practise independently or pose a risk to patient/client safety. Again, this decision could not be taken in isolation and needs to be informed by the expert opinion of others, for example occupational health and/or a doctor.

How supported are students with disabilities at university?

All universities will have a dedicated centre for student support services, often including staff employed purely to support the needs of disabled students. As part of the application process, you may well have already contacted these services – to help you maximise the support on offer during selection days for example. Once you're on the programme, it's highly recommended that you don't struggle alone or underestimate the impact that your new life may have on your health. It is wise therefore, to make early and regular contact. This is to ensure that you receive as much advice and support as possible while at university, and also to make a plan for the specific areas of support that you may need while working in clinical practice. Here is one example of how to cope with the demands of the course if you are a student with dyslexia.

Suzanne Lloyd, Second-year Midwifery Student

I have been dyslexic all my life. I suffered at the hands of school bullies and teachers that just didn't understand that a dyslexic person is as bright and intelligent as anyone else. I did not get the results at GCSE that I had hoped for and truly feel that this was because of the lack of help, support and understanding received at school. Yet here I am now, at the age of 34, half-way through a BSc Hons Midwifery degree and fulfilling a dream that I never thought possible.

When I came to look at what help and support my university would/could give a dyslexic person I was stunned for all the right reasons. I have one-to-one help for an hour a week which is just amazing. My support worker is always happy to help; she reads all my work and helps with the grammar and spelling side of things. She will not change the content but she will tell me 'what did you mean – that sentence makes no sense'. The course is very hard work, and not just for a dyslexic person. I have to be very organised which can be especially hard. However, the motivation to succeed is what keeps me going.

As part of my NHS bursary I get financial help so that meant I could buy a laptop with all the additional software included to specifically help me. I find that reading is hard when it is black on white – so I have a program that will change the colour of the screen which makes the reading a bit easier! Reading is a big part of the course, and all my friends sit around talking about what they read last night, just for 'fun'. I don't have this luxury – it takes all my time to read what is needed to get through the course. Now my friends will tell me more so that I don't need to read the entire book, and if the item is of real interest they will tell me which part to read.

I thought that when I got to university, I would leave all the bullying about dyslexia behind me – this hasn't always been the case. Although I have a good group of friends that have helped and supported me, some students don't understand that dyslexia doesn't automatically equate with low intelligence. Comments such as 'I want to work with someone who will bring my grades up', or 'You're dyslexic – I need help but not from you', can be very hurtful and reveal the lack of knowledge people have about dyslexia, as well as other learning needs. My support worker has been very helpful, as have the university tutors. I feel that I am doing much better than ever I thought I would. When I started the course my plan was to pass, but most of my grades have been 'C' and above. Now that I know I can do it and have had a taste of a 'B+', I am aiming for my first 'A'.

In the practice setting, things have been easier. I have always been forthcoming and told my mentors, as there are a lot of notes that must be written correctly and legibly – again this is a challenge for the dyslexic, especially as record-keeping must be done at the same time as care is given. With the help and understanding of two senior midwives who gave me so much of their time, my confidence has now grown with the notes.

Here are my top tips for successful studying with dyslexia:

- Tell people that you have dyslexia. Be proud of it and hold your head up high, because if we don't, the stigma will remain and nothing will change.

- I have a 'cheat sheet' in my bag so that when I am writing the notes, I can see that what is written is different from what we say, and also to check correct spellings. For example, we might say 'listening in to baby', but we write 'auscultating the fetal heart'. I don't need the sheet as much as I did, but it's good to know it is there as a 'back up', especially when I'm tired at the end of a long shift.

- For the university work you need to be organised – file the paperwork as soon as you get home! With written assignments, I always consider that the submission date is four weeks before it actually is. This gives me lots of precious time – to get the work to my tutor to look at and feedback comments and make any changes that are needed. Then I still have two weeks for my dyslexia support worker to check the grammar and spelling.

- We all have our own coping strategies but it is important to have them in place at the very start when you are doing such an intensive course like nursing or midwifery.

- Lastly, have good support at home from friends and family. Although I don't see them as much as I would like, when you have had a hard day at university or on the wards, a hug can really help.

Remember that just because you are dyslexic does not mean 'you can't' – it just means you may have to try a bit harder, but it can be done and I still love my course as much as I did at the start.

Summary

- Ensure that you have confidently chosen the right career path *before* applying. Admissions tutors only have limited places to offer and are therefore looking for applicants who have a very good understanding of their nursing field of practice, or midwifery.

- Completion of the personal statement is key to being shortlisted and is therefore a task that requires planning, practice and support – do not underestimate this task.

- Remember to state not only *what* you know about your chosen profession, but also *how* you know.

- Selection days are highly stressful for candidates – they require planning, preparation and practice.

- First impressions count – remember to SMILE.

- Applicants who have a disability, or past caution/conviction, are not automatically excluded from the professions. Systems are in place to help support the needs of such candidates – early disclosure is key to accessing this support and therefore maximising the likelihood of success.

- Remember that courses such as child health nursing and midwifery are heavily oversubscribed. This makes the competition for places tough and if you are not successful at the first attempt, reflect on the feedback given and try again next year.

Interview checklist

University	
Course title	
Personal University Reference #	
UCAS #	
Dates/notes of contacts:	Dates/times/method (phone, email). Keep hard copies of any emails or letters.
Date of interview	
Venue	
Time:	To: From:
Contact	Name: Phone: Email:
Documents required for interview	Originals of identification and education documents

	Are copies needed? Y/N How many? Copies made (date)
What test/s will be used?	Details
Key names/contacts	
Travel arrangements, times, cost	
Who have I told where I am going?	Tell at least one person where you are going/when you will be back, and leave them a copy of your travel plans and interview details.
Useful information/notes	
When will I hear back?	University's decision
My ranking of the course	My decision

Selection day resources

http://www.mymathlab.com/global
MyMathLab is an online practice and assessment resource that comes with the textbook, *Numeracy in Nursing and Healthcare*, Pearl Shihab (2010), Harlow: Pearson Education (ISBN 978-14-0826851-3).

Brilliant Interview (3rd edn) Ros Jay (2010), Harlow: Pearson Education (978-0-273-74393-4)

http://www.bbc.co.uk/skillswise/
Resources to help develop basic English and Maths skills.

http://labspace.open.ac.uk/
Higher education learning resources.

http://www.learnhigher.ac.uk/home.html
Resources that help students with a range of higher education skills.

http://www.lsbu.ac.uk/hsc/courses/interviews.shtml#tests
Examples of numeracy and literacy tests for nursing/midwifery used at London South Bank University.

http://www.testandcalc.com/
Drug calculation resources for healthcare professionals.

http://www.thestudentroom.co.uk/
Advice and resources for university students, including preparation for interviews.

http://www.studentmidwife.net/
Education-based site for student midwives and applicants to midwifery programmes.

http://www.studentnurse.org.uk/
Education-based site for student nurses and applicants to nursing programmes.

http://www.uwl.ac.uk/nursing/faq/quiz.jsp
Example of numeracy test for nursing used at University of West London.

Interview survival kit

- Spare tights/stockings (if applicable)
- Hairbrush/comb
- Deodorant
- Mouth freshener/mints
- House/car keys
- Smart bag with sufficient space to accommodate everything
- Umbrella
- Travel pass etc.
- A watch
- Copy of UCAS application
- Academic certificates
- Pens, pencils, eraser, ruler and calculator (you will normally not be allowed to use your mobile phone)
- Any sports kit if doing fitness test
- Plasters – you may be doing a lot of walking
- Paracetamol
- Tissues
- Useful phone numbers (in case your phone goes flat)
- Spot concealer/makeup
- Loose change
- Emergency cash/credit card
- Mobile phone (fully charged with good amount of credit)
- Consider a mobile phone charger
- Something to read
- Any research notes you have made on key topics
- Map
- Photographic ID/document e.g. driving license, passport. You may be asked to prove your identity
- Interview invitation letter
- Cash for lunch/drinks/car parks

Sample interview questions

- How do you feel the day has gone so far?
- How can the NHS provide a more cost-effective service to patients who are chronically ill?
- What qualities do you feel make a successful nurse*?
- What is the role of health promotion?
- Why do you want to become an adult/child/mental health nurse?
- Team working is important; can you give me an example of how you work in teams?
- Tell me about a time when you have faced a problem? How did you overcome this?
- How do you think your tutor/a colleague would describe you?
- You will need to start work at 7.00 a.m, may finish late at night, and be required to work night shifts. How do you think this will affect your life?
- Describe a stressful situation you have experienced.
- How will you support yourself financially while at university?
- How do you keep fit?
- If you were given £1 million today what would you spend this on in the NHS and why?
- What worries you most about working in healthcare?
- What do you think are the main health challenges facing the NHS today/in the future?
- What research have you done into nursing careers?
- Tell me about your work experience.
- What would you do if a patient told you they were thinking of killing themselves?

*Substitute your chosen profession. 'Nurse/nursing' has been used as an example.

Chapter 4

Pre-course preparation

Learning outcomes

By the end of Chapter 4, you should be able to:

- ✔ obtain a realistic picture of the imminent demands that will be placed on you as a healthcare student, and feel more confident to meet them
- ✔ identify some of the practical strategies that can be put in place to help smooth the transition to the higher education environment
- ✔ consider the importance of emotional intelligence in supporting your personal and professional development
- ✔ look forward to the beginning of your new career
- ✔ locate some of the pre-course reading material suggested to help prepare for life-long learning

Introduction

This chapter shifts the focus to the time leading up to the start date of your nursing and midwifery programme. It is based on some practical suggestions that address important issues in your life that can perhaps be organised, or at least considered, during this precious window of time. This advice is drawn from a rich pot of experience – that of teaching staff, mentors and students.

Start-up skills

Congratulations! You've worked extremely hard to arrive at this point; prepared extensively, performed very well at selection point, and been offered a place. This is a very significant achievement and you are quite right to be delighted. You're now well on the way to securing your goal of being a registered nurse or midwife, and probably the weeks or months before your start date can't pass quickly enough. So, how will you spend your time? Taking it easy and relaxing? Wrong! This precious window of time is the perfect opportunity to prepare your life, and the lives of your family, which will never be the same again. Use this time wisely and you will reap the benefits later on when they are needed most.

As you read this chapter, consider Box 4.1 which lists the key student survival attributes, recently canvassed from a group of first-year student nurses. They might help put this chapter into clearer context, as well as emphasise that the suggestions contained within it are actually quite a good idea.

> ## Box 4.1 Student survival attributes
>
> 1. Organisational skills
> 2. Determination to succeed
> 3. Seek support – from tutors, family, friends, fellow students, mentors
> 4. Commitment
> 5. Motivation

The chapter now looks in detail at practical ways to prepare for your studies to come.

 ## Save money

You won't be rich as a student nurse/midwife. At the moment, an income-assessed bursary is the entitlement for students on undergraduate programmes, but it is just that – means tested. This means that the assessment is based on your entire household's income, not just your own. Many undergraduate nursing and midwifery students receive little in the way of a bursary and often struggle to make ends meet, especially if they have taken the plunge and left home. You will read one student's advice about managing this in Chapter 5. Many students report that they have waited months for their bursary to arrive, therefore apply for it as soon as your place is confirmed.

It therefore makes good sense to save as much money as you can during the time that you are waiting to start your training programme, and think about ways that you can minimise start-up costs. If you're moving into rented accommodation, start acquiring the items you'll need to make it your home and therefore a refuge from the demands of the programme. Don't rush out and buy lots of books that will then spend three years sitting on the shelf. Remember that there will probably be only a few key texts that you will need to purchase, and those can usually be bought cheaply second hand, through Amazon for example. Many universities run second hand book schemes too. Plan your birthday and Christmas present lists wisely!

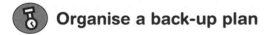 ## Organise a back-up plan

It's very difficult to appreciate the rigours of shift work unless you've actually done it. Remember that the nature of your profession may mean staying over your shifts at times – babies won't be born to your timeframe; transferring a patient to a specialist unit can significantly delay you getting home. University time is far more easily managed because the teaching day is generally based around the hours of a 'normal' working day. However, half of the course will be spent in clinical practice and that means shift work around the clock, so think about who you're going to rely on when you want to be there at that baby's birth; support that patient as he is transferred to a specialist unit for treatment that could save his life. When you've arranged that back-up person, then sort out another one, so you eventually have a chain of trusted people that you can rely on to help you out when life in practice becomes complicated. When you're busy in the clinical environments, and know that you're going to be late and can't pick up your children from school, all you'll be able to manage is a quick text to your back-up team. This plan is particularly important during school holidays, as you must not rely on your university course holidays matching them.

Thinking ahead is the key to minimising your stress and practising your back-up system before you arrive at university is extremely wise. Even if you don't have dependants, you still need to plan ahead. For example, when your flatmates plan a night out when you're in the middle of placement, you'll need to remind them that you'll be asleep in bed when they return late, and going to work very early the next morning.

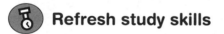 Refresh study skills

Most university entrance requirements demand evidence of recent study, as they know that academic life can be rather a shock for people who have been away from it for some time. However, it's easy to become 'rusty' after even a relatively short time, so consider how you will keep your intellectual skills ticking over, ready for the start of the programme. Your university will probably have sent you some pre-course reading to consider, so this is an excellent first starting point. Pre-course reading does not mean attempting to digest an entire textbook – you'll quickly become bored and overwhelmed, so try different options first. As relevant anatomy and physiology will feature early on in your nursing or midwifery programme, it makes good sense to read around the body systems, and there are lots of innovative resources available that make this a very manageable task.

At the end of this chapter you'll find a list of 'friendly' resources that will launch your career as a life-long learner. Smaller libraries probably won't stock the books and journals, so you'll need to visit to a bigger one, or try your local university's library – many are open to the public but may have restricted borrowing rights. The key with reading is quality, not quantity. There's no point at all in devouring an entire reading list if at the end of it you can't recall any significant issues from the texts. The ability to retain and then recall such information is a key academic skill, so be discerning from the very beginning. Also try to keep a summary of each book, journal and website that you read, known as an annotated bibliography. A template for creating a basic bibliography has been provided for you at the end of the chapter (see p. 113). Compiling this type of summary is a very valuable academic skill that you will apply early on in your programme, so practise it now. You'll then have made a great start at developing your organisational and recall skills.

If it is a long time since you've used a computer regularly, or you're not well practised at certain applications, now is a good time to embrace the technology on offer. Like it or not, universities will utilise a range of web-based learning as part of the course and require written assessments to be word-processed. Many colleges run evening classes to help people brush up on their IT skills, often for a very modest fee, so if you're feeling anxious about the whole concept, investigate such classes and try out your skills. Of course, you'll be helped and supported once you start university – it's just a huge boost to your confidence if you understand the principles of some of the technology on offer before you actually arrive. The range of skills that you'll be expected to use during your course include some or all of the following:

- Submitting written work as a word-processed document, usually Microsoft Word; using a package such as PowerPoint for presentations.
- Searching the Internet for articles and information via university accessed databases.
- Using email to contact peers and tutors; posting to blogs and websites.
- Accessing dedicated websites for student information, assessment results, course information etc.
- Engaging with virtual learning environments.

ometimes, electronic learning also involves the use of social networking sites such as Facebook. However, approach this with caution as
the type of material you will post within the context of your course will
be profoundly different from that posted as part of your social life. Once
you start university, clear guidelines will be issued to you about professional boundaries and the type of information not to include in such
sites. As a general rule, do not disclose *any* information about clients or
patients, university staff, other students, or hospital Trusts/staff that
is likely to cause offence. Any disclosure that results in a breach of
confidentiality is a very serious matter, and will involve professional
conduct review at either university or NMC level. It is therefore important that you quickly familiarise yourself with safe and professional
conduct when using social networking sites, for example by reviewing
the guidance provided by the NMC on their website (**www.nmc-uk.org**).

Health and well-being

The demands made upon you once you start the course can seem
relentless at times. Remember that nursing and midwifery are physically and emotionally demanding occupations where you'll be on your
feet for long periods of time and dealing with people experiencing
high levels of stress. All this, together with erratic breaks when on
placement, shift work, and assessment load, can generate periods
of intense stress for students. Sometimes, this stress can become
unbearable and result in students temporarily 'stepping' off their
course or even leaving it altogether. These important issues, and
the resilience required to cope with them are explored in more detail
in Chapter 5. Meanwhile, there are a number of strategies that you
can employ to prepare yourself for the demands of the course, not
least amongst them improving your overall fitness and good health.
It is estimated that during each 12-hour shift, nurses walk 4–5 miles
(Welton et al, 2006). Imagine doing that every day for a week and
how tired you'll become. So, although I don't suggest you develop a
passion for mountain climbing or marathon running during the time
period before you start your course, it is good to think about getting
fitter. If you've been planning to quit smoking, reduce the amount
of alcohol you drink, or lose some weight, the start date of a course

can be an excellent motivator. Moderating our habits and being more physically active every day is good for all of us. For student nurses and midwives, it can be key to resilience during times of acute stress, as well as providing an excellent health promotion opportunity for the people you come into contact with every day. A pregnant woman who is obese is more likely to listen to a midwife who shares her own experience of losing weight; a nurse promoting smoking cessation will probably gain more respect if her clients know that she has successfully stopped smoking herself.

 ## Emotional intelligence

The concept of emotional intelligence (EI) is not new, but is now increasingly being applied to an understanding of the high order skills required of nurses and midwives in their daily practice. It has been defined as 'the subset of social intelligence that involves the ability to monitor one's own and others' feelings and emotions, to discriminate among them and to use this information to guide one's thinking and actions' (Salovey and Mayer, 1990).

There are many tests available that assess your EI, similar to those used to measure IQ. People who have a high EI score tend to demonstrate skills related to the understanding and interpretation of emotions, as well as the best way to act upon them. There are clear links with these and the skills required of a reflective practitioner, an ability that will also be required of you during the development of your career as a nurse or midwife. People who practice EI are skilled at dealing with social or emotional conflict, can freely express their emotions, and are able to manage them through a variety of life experiences (Goleman, 1995).

You may consider that it is impossible to learn the skills of reflection and EI - surely they must be innate? There is much current debate about this, especially in relation to the practice of healthcare professionals, but it may be that such skills are not impossible to develop or refine over time. A recent *Sunday Times* article highlighted the work being done by Professor VS Ramachandran, a scientist researching the amazing capacity of the human brain to change. We therefore cannot dismiss an individual's ability to foster new skills, given that our understanding of the human brain is still in its relative infancy.

As an imminent student nurse or midwife, it would be beneficial to think about the concept of emotional intelligence in terms of your own journey to this point. Did you, for example, perhaps not obtain a place on your course at the first attempt? Rather than give up, or look to someone else to blame, did you instead reflect on the experience, consider the feedback that was given to you, and make a plan to improve and try again? If so, that would suggest that you have EI in abundance and will be able to apply the same reasoning behaviour to the range of emotional situations soon to be encountered. If you know from other experiences that you have some work to do yet in managing your emotional life, then try out some strategies now – just by thinking about them is a good start to develop your EI and can only benefit your experiences as a student.

TOP TIPS

- *Remind everyone close to you about the demands that you're about to face when joining the course, especially the people you love – they will face their own challenges when the person they love seems to have temporarily disappeared out of their life.*

- *Prime your sense of humour – you're going to need it.*

- *Learn to drive and borrow or buy a car. Not all clinical placements can be accessed using public transport, especially rural ones, and the more independent you are as a student, the more you will be able to access the full range of available learning opportunities, for example attending a homebirth in the middle of the night, or arranging an elective placement in a regional transplant unit some miles from your 'home' university. I have very fond memories of getting around on a pushbike in my first year as a student midwife – I've never been so fit!*

- *Plan ahead as much as you can, and anticipate some of the demands that will occur within your non-student nurse/midwife life, for example school holiday cover.*

- *Rest, relax and look forward to a rollercoaster ride of experiences – hopefully more 'ups' than 'downs'.*

Summary

- The period of time between obtaining a place on a healthcare course and starting it can be equally exciting and anxiety-provoking. This is entirely normal.

- The practical advice and suggestions contained within this chapter should help alleviate some of this anxiety through enabling you to plan and prepare.

- The concept of emotional intelligence is important to the experience of healthcare students because of the nature of the professions, and the consequential demands made upon student nurses and midwives.

- Pre-course reading is an important first step in your journey as a life-long learner. Remember that this reading is about quality, not quantity.

Friendly pre-course reading

This is not an exhaustive list, rather a selection of books, websites and journals that will be of interest to you and they have been chosen to appeal to a broad range of abilities. A good starting point would be to view the web resources – they are free, easy to access and contain an excellent range of information, most of which you can download easily. The university will send you their own list of pre-course reading once your place is confirmed – the following are just suggestions to start you off in the meantime.

Nursing & Health Survival Guides – this pocket-sized series is available at all good bookshops and online and covers a wide range of topics including Clnical Skills, Maths and Medications, Clinical Abbreviations and Normal Values, Compassion, Caring and Communication, OSCE tests, Health Promotion, Nutrition and Hydration, Midwifery Skills and much more.

Bach S and Grant A (2009), *Communication and Interpersonal Skills for Nurses*. Southernhay: Learning Matters.

Bloomfield et al (2010), *How to Pass Your OSCE*. Harlow: Pearson Education.

Burnard P and Gill P (2009), *Culture, Communication and Nursing*. Harlow: Pearson Education.

Colbert et al (2012), *Anatomy & Physiology for Nursing & Healthcare*. Harlow: Pearson Education.

Department of Health: http://www.dh.gov.uk/en/index.htm

Foss M and Farine T (2008), *Science in Nursing & Healthcare*. Harlow: Pearson Education.

Garret et al (2011), *Skills for Nursing & Healthcare Students: Study Skills, Maths and Science*. Harlow: Pearson Education.

Health Information Resources: http://www.library.nhs.uk/default.aspx

Johnson R and Taylor W (2006), *Skills for Midwifery Practice*. Edinburgh: Churchill Livingstone.

Jolley J (2010), *Introducing Research and Evidence-based Practice for Nurses*. Harlow: Pearson Education.

Kirkham M (ed) (2010), *The Midwife–Mother Relationship*. New York: Palgrave Macmillan.

Kozier et al (2012), *Fundamentals of Nursing* (2nd edn). Harlow: Pearson Education.

LearnHigher: http://www.learnhigher.ac.uk/students.htm

Maier P, Price G and Cowen M (2009), *Study Skills for Nursing and Healthcare Students*. Harlow: Pearson Education.

Mander R and Fleming V (eds) (2009), *Becoming a Midwife*. Abingdon: Routledge.

Marieb EN and Hoehn K (2009), *Human Anatomy & Physiology with Interactive Physiology 10 System Suite*. London: Benjamin Cummings.

National Institute for Health and Clinical Excellence: http://www.nice.org.uk/

Nursing Times: http://info.nursingtimes.net/

Olsen et al (2010), *Dosage Calculations for Nurses*. Harlow: Pearson Education.

The Practising Midwife: http://www.practisingmidwife.co.uk/

Sellman D and Snelling P (2009), *Becoming a Nurse*. Harlow: Pearson Education.

Shihab P (2010), *Numeracy in Nursing and Healthcare plus MyMathLab*. Harlow: Pearson Education.

Siviter B (2008), *The Student Nurse Handbook*. Edinburgh: Baillière Tindall.

Smith B and Field L (2011), *Nursing Care*. Harlow: Pearson Education.

World Health Organization: http://www.who.int/en/

Wylie L (2005), *Essential Anatomy and Physiology in Maternity Care*. Edinburgh: Churchill Livingstone.

Annotated bibliography tool

1. Full reference of book/article/website:

2. What the resource is about:

3. Why I liked it:

4. What I didn't like about it:

5. How I think it will help me as a student nurse or midwife:

Chapter 5

Planning for adversity: building resilience

Learning outcomes

By the end of Chapter 5, you should be able to:

✔ consider the particular anxieties of 'mature' students, and how these might be addressed
✔ identify some of the reasons students leave their courses early
✔ reflect on the characteristics of students most likely to complete their courses
✔ identify strategies that can support resilience in healthcare students and encourage them to stay

Introduction

Well done for reaching the end of the book - your head must now be completely full of information. At this stage, we need to think a little more about the realities of life as a student nurse or midwife. As you have no doubt realised by now, this career choice is not to be taken lightly as the demands involved are intense. Many students find these demands exceed their capabilities or expectations and make a painful decision to leave. For everyone involved, this represents a significant loss and is one therefore to be minimised. This final chapter will address these issues in more detail, and is drawn from the contributions of people who have experienced at first hand what you're about to experience, or who have accrued many years of expertise in supporting students through a period of transition.

 ## Older and wiser

Martin Spurin

Oh my God! What am I doing? Going to university at my time of life? I'll never be able to do it. I wasn't particularly that good at school. I didn't even like school. Everyone else in my group will be okay; it will just be me who doesn't understand. I'm not sure if my writing is that good – not at this level. Higher education? That can't be for me, can it?

Returning to education as an adult can be quite daunting. If you've said any of the above statements then you are not alone. In fact, nearly everyone in your group will be feeling exactly the same. The first day is probably the worst. You're entering a new building, being put with new people who will be your fellow students for the next couple of years and then you've got to meet those academic lecturers...worse still, they also happen to be very experienced nurses and midwives and they're going to give you loads of work to do.

This all sounds a bit negative, but in actual fact as an adult you have such an advantage over students who come straight from school. You have experience. You have opinions. You have knowledge of what it's like in the real world. You've worked; you've worked with people – and some strange people at that – you've worked for managers, good ones and bad ones. Quite possibly, you've worked within the Health Service and already engaged with caring for others. You've evaluated what it was like to be treated as an employee. Young students rarely have this abundance of experience and therefore a lot of what is taught can mean so little to them at times. Teaching adults like you is great because of what you can bring and the contribution you can make.

Do you get the impression that going to lectures at university means sitting in a large lecture theatre listening to someone who seems very detached from you and is speaking above your head? That might happen occasionally if you're unlucky, but generally most classes can be very interactive. Most tutors welcome contributions from students and encourage discussion, especially when it's about patient care. Don't be afraid to ask questions in class especially if you don't understand something. You might notice the relief on your fellow students' faces when you do that, because very often if you don't understand something you can guarantee others don't understand it either, but they're afraid to speak up. Confidence in adults as students can be very fragile and brittle at times and they may need someone like you to help them voice their concerns.

Most understand what it's like for you returning to education. They realise that your priorities lie elsewhere, namely: first, family; second, clinical practice; and third, university. Don't lose sight of this too. Your family has to come first as that is probably the most important thing in your life. With placements, you have obligations and responsibilities that you must achieve (and usually enjoy). University usually comes third on the list, and perhaps rightly so. The problem you'll face is that at times you'll feel as though it's impossible to cope with it all and that everything is becoming too much. This can often be the case especially as terms (or semesters as they're usually called now) are often quite short and thus, very intense. Assignments pile up, deadlines get closer and you will feel as though it's all getting on top of you. But you are not alone – everyone else is feeling the same too.

Why does it have to be so intense? Well, as you've found out from other chapters in this book professional courses make huge demands on the development of your academic and clinical practice skills in a relatively short space of time. Sometimes, shorter programmes are an option, for example if you are already a graduate and seeking to apply for nursing. Two years spent following this route seems much easier to cope with and make a commitment to than three years, therefore the weeks that you are in university will be quite intense. But don't forget that some annual leave and independent study is part of the course too! There are 52 weeks in a year and your course probably runs for about 45 weeks of the year.

One thing you'll also find is that you'll start off keeping up with everything, you might even find things are not too bad and feel excited that at long last, you're actually caring for people in clinical practice instead of just talking about it – but then you'll hit a plateau. This is a phase that most students go through. It's a phase when things are getting a bit harder, it's all becoming rather difficult and you'll question yourself whether it's all worth it. You may have received a grade for a piece of work, which you were very disappointed with (and one you had spent many hours on as well), or have worked with a mentor less helpful than the previous one. You question whether it's worth continuing because you just don't feel up to it. This is the plateau! This is when students generally tend to think about leaving a course. But if you can, just be aware of it, accept that it's a natural part of your course, and others will reach the same point. It's part of being a student again. If you can persevere you'll find that after a few weeks you'll start to realise your own progress as well as the potential you have. It's not that 'you don't get it' – it's because you've entered a new world, a different world to the one you feel comfortable in. This is where a reflective diary can be so helpful – reading back on your experience within the first clinical placement for example, will illuminate just how far you've travelled.

The problem is that we don't notice our own progress because it's so gradual and we're very critical of ourselves. We do expect a lot from ourselves and this stems from the fear of failure. How do we identify our progress? One way of doing this is by looking at a piece of work that you did about 18 months ago. Very often you'll see that your writing has developed without you noticing. There are two reasons for this: first, you've had feedback on your assignments which you have taken into consideration when you've approached other pieces of work; and second, it takes practice to write essays and reports in an academic way. Don't feel that you've got to get it right straight away. Yes there will be students who will get high grades right from the beginning and find it all so easy – but they're in the minority, so don't compare yourself with them. Compare yourself to the majority of students who are like you. To be honest, you should make all your mistakes in your first year – that's why first-year grades don't contribute to your final classification. As long as you are using the feedback to develop and you are learning, then you're making progress.

On most courses you'll attend classes and go home and may not return for several weeks, especially when on placement, so most of the time you'll be on your own. Your priorities then, as regards your coursework, are the assignments. Don't feel you have to understand everything that is covered in classes. It's the assignments that you need to concentrate on, as it's these that determine whether you get through the course or not. It's these that demonstrate your understanding. That's why it can be really useful finding out whether there is anyone in your group who lives near you. It can make it so much easier if you can spend time with someone in your group, share ideas and just have someone to bounce ideas off.

The one thing that most current students advise new students is to start assignments early to give yourself enough opportunity to make changes and redraft. Lizzie identifies this clearly in Reflection 5.1. If you leave things to nearer the deadline it becomes very stressful and pressurised. If you have an essay to write, it's always advisable to make a plan of the essay before you start and check with your tutor (or the person marking it) to see whether you are on the right track. It is so easy to drift away from the question asked in the assignment and many students do this. Keep in mind that you can only get marks if you answer the question that has been set. It's also a good idea to ask your tutor if you can look at previous examples of work that other students have done. You may not be shown really good pieces of work because your tutor may not want you to feel that you can't reach those heights, not at this stage anyway, but he or she could show you elements of good and poor pieces of work. So do ask – what have you got to lose?

TOP TIPS

- Start your work early; don't leave it to the last moment - not at this level.

- Do a plan of your work and show it to your tutor to see whether you're on the right track.

- I know academics will look down on this, but if you're struggling with a topic and you want to have a basic understanding of it look at something like Wikipedia. Get an understanding and then look at your recommended reading (but don't use Wikipedia in your work - just use it to get you going).

- Don't expect too much from yourself - especially in the first year. It takes practise writing well and it takes a while to get used to this new level of study.

- Referencing - this can be quite hard to get used to, so don't expect to get this right straight away (some academics still get it wrong).

- Find a study buddy, someone who lives near you so you can work together and support each other.

- If possible, redistribute jobs at home so that you can have more time, and if possible schedule blocks of time for you (that's if you can retrain the family at home).

- Remember you have rights as a student, so if you don't feel that the quality of your provision is satisfactory then you should speak up - otherwise nothing will ever change. If there were no students like you there would be no need for the staff.

- Hang in there when things seem to be getting tough - remember everyone goes through this. Use the support facilities; they are there for you, but if you don't use them or tell someone you need help, how can they start to reach you? Don't lose sight of your original motivation to enter a healthcare profession.

- Be committed even before you start. Make sure that this is for you and this is what you want. Set realistic goals for yourself and start ticking them off as you reach them.

And one last thing - read this chapter at least once a month just to put things into perspective - it will make you feel better.

From a student's point of view

Lizzie Hilliard, Finalist Student Midwife

From an early age (about 7 years old), I had shown an unrealised interest in midwifery, as I played with my dolls wearing a dressing-up nurse's outfit. A few years later, my understanding about midwifery was established and from the moment I knew what a midwife did, I aspired to be one. When I was 14 years old, I worked hard at school to gain good SATs results, as I already knew that I required excellent grades to step into a midwifery career. During this year, I accompanied my older brother to attend an open day at Worcester University, at which I persuaded my parents to visit the midwifery area. I was so excited. Upon entering the room, I spoke to a male lecturer, who tried to influence me to become a nurse - but no! I knew the career path I had to pursue. He advised me to read midwifery journals, which I did. I don't know what this lecturer thought of me, a 14-year-old girl! Following this, I found out about the Midwifery taster days, which Worcester University ran, so I contacted the appropriate person and was lucky enough to be allocated a place for this day. I was 15 years old then and I took as much information on board as possible, so I had an understanding of what to do when I applied for a University place. After my GCSEs, I completed a few voluntary placements, including the following:

- I spent an afternoon with a community midwife at a group for pregnant women;

- I completed work experience in a nursery baby unit to learn how to care for babies;

- I went to a nursing home to get experience with caring for adults (this was encouraged);

- I spent a week with a health visitor;

● After a long time of arranging, I managed to set up a week's placement at Birmingham Women's Hospital, seeing both antenatal and postnatal wards.

These experiences reinforced that midwifery was definitely the right career for me. Following them, I studied appropriate 'A' Levels which would support my application to the midwifery course (Biology, Psychology, Health and Social Care, General Studies and an AS in Philosophy and Ethics). During the second year of completing my 'A' Levels, I received advice and submitted my personal statement to Worcester University. After receiving an offer of an interview, I knew I was one step closer to becoming a student midwife. All I had to do now was to pull off a good interview. I researched recent articles, practised my maths (for the maths test), made my mum listen to me rehearsing interviews and bought a new suit. Just over a week after the interview, I received a 'conditional' offer from Worcester University and was ecstatic. The next hurdle was passing my 'A' Levels, which thankfully I did and now knew I was definitely going to be a student midwife! All the determination of the past few years was starting to pay off.

During my first year as a student midwife, I studied at university combined with placements in the community, labour ward and postnatal ward. I enjoyed all these placements, despite being anxious about what I was going to see at the start. However, all my mentors were lovely and very supportive. The first birth I witnessed was in the community, a homebirth that was absolutely amazing. This was also the first time I actually had my hands on at a birth and that was completely overwhelming and unforgettable. Since then, I have helped deliver 19 babies and each event has been wonderfully different. Prior to each new birth, it is true to say that the unexpected has to be expected. This creates an unbelievable excitement, which can only be experienced as a student midwife and makes all the ups and downs, also experienced, completely worthwhile. For me, this also became a survival tool and encouraged my continued enthusiasm for this career. Some of the placements I completed did not initially appear to link to midwifery, especially in my second year when, for instance, I undertook placements on the gynaecology ward and Critical Care Unit. However, I now appreciate that these placements have been incorporated into the midwifery programme as they do have a purpose in educating students about the care of critically ill people, as this may be relevant to future midwifery situations. Embracing these placements with an open mind and a friendly attitude certainly helped to widen my knowledge and understanding. Experiencing some unfortunate and sad occasions during training has helped me to accept that there are such times, and by taking up offers of support from others, i.e. mentors, colleagues and family, has strengthened my approach to deal with future events.

I am now well into my final year – scary! But also very exciting. There is even more academic work, for instance the independent study, together with lengthier placements. However, being completely honest, I cannot wait to finish this year and fulfil my lifelong aspiration to become a registered midwife. I am pleased that communicating with people at all levels has become more practised and hopefully this will be an aid during my final year. My enthusiasm, determination and interest remains and I hope to survive this year by sustaining a positive and friendly attitude.

Reflecting on my past years and especially the last two, I would suggest to any student midwife to embrace all opportunities, even if you are not keen on them, as another placement will soon arise, so accept it, learn from it, smile and enjoy it! There are a few skills and attributes that student nurses and midwives should have or master, so I have put together some 'Survival Tips' that may help some students during their nursing or midwifery courses, and they are as follows:

1. Dedication – having a passion for caring for people. In midwifery, this is antepartum/intrapartum/postpartum women, their babies and families.

2. Flexibility – you will be on different shift/hours while on placement combined with lots of university work, e.g. portfolios, presentations and essays.

3. Realise – that this is a hard course. When you get in from night shifts and have university work on your mind and you're tired, just think of your end goal – all the hard work will pay off.

4. Young students – living at home is probably best. That's what I have found, as it's much cheaper and you are probably more likely to receive support from parents and friends.

5. Mums – there are lots of mums in my cohort; make sure your kids come first! Accept help from friends and families – you will value their support.

6. Smile – it makes all the difference; it is contagious.

7. Learn and accept that all criticism equals a positive! Receive as much support from tutors as possible to aim higher with academic work.

8. Respect – clinicians, mentors, other health professionals, lecturers and other students – they will all help you at some point.

9. Always look for the strengths in placement, situations, academic work and people in general; you will be a happier student midwife. Turn the negatives into positives, talk to other students, tutors and family about your problems – it *always* helps.

10. Communication – this skill is a *must*! Always think about what you are going to say and force yourself to practise – it's the only way forward.

11. The three 'Ps' – be **p**roactive, **p**lan ahead and **p**rioritise – combining all three 'Ps' will enable essential organisation of academic work and placements.

12. Embrace all placements and get as much out of them as you can!

Remember these 'Survival Tips' and hopefully you will enjoy and succeed in your nursing or midwifery course. Good luck!

🔖 The successful student

Kim Russell

By the time you read this chapter you will understand some of the joys and difficulties others have encountered on their journey to achieve their goal of being a professional nurse or midwife. For these reasons I decided to use the analogy of Tolkien's *Lord of the Rings* to convey the intensity and unpredictable nature of professional degree programmes and that the positive and negative experiences you will have along the way will be transformational. I am not saying that you will have to climb mountains and fight evil, but like Frodo Baggins you will face life changing events that will push you to the limit of your intellectual and physical abilities. As you will have already gleaned from this chapter, the majority of students are successful in their studies because they have been able to negotiate any barriers to study through careful planning and by being highly motivated individuals.

The aim of this section is to provide you with a metaphorical rucksack of survival tips to guide you through the first year of study and beyond. At the start of your journey you will need a clear understanding of some of the problems other nursing and midwifery students have faced. You can then take preventative steps to avoid discontinuing your journey before qualification.

Planning for adversity: starting out

In a study by Yorke and Longden (2008), first-year degree students on non-professional degree courses gave the following reasons for discontinuing their studies:

- poor-quality learning experiences (16.6 per cent);
- not coping with academic demand (9.6 per cent);
- wrong choice of course (8.7 per cent);
- unhappy with the location of the university and environment (7.0 per cent);
- dissatisfied with institutional resources (6.8 per cent);
- problems with finance (6.3 per cent);
- problems with making friends and social engagement (5.9 per cent).

This research found that first-year undergraduates were more likely to leave university during breaks between semesters or at holiday times (Easter and Christmas). Unhappiness with the course, problems with making friends, 'fitting in' and home sickness appear to be the reasons for this type of behaviour. These students tended to be under 26 years of age, living in rented accommodation and studying modular degrees on a full- or part-time basis. The main reasons given by first-year nursing students on the other hand were failure in academic and/or clinical assessments and personal problems (Deary et al, 2003). Personal problems included financial worries, family or relationship problems, and physical or psychological sickness. It appears that students on nursing and midwifery courses suffer higher levels of stress and burnout than students on traditional degree programmes because of the need to work shifts and study on a full-time basis (Deary et al, 2003; Green and Baird, 2009). Students who fail to manage their stress levels are less likely to cope with the demands placed upon them and more likely to leave their courses before reaching the third year. Interestingly, higher levels of stress appear to be associated with clinical practice placements. Time spent in university appears to be less stressful because of the support offered by academic staff and fellow students. Midwifery students who had an unrealistic view of the role of the midwife, the demands of midwifery practice (emotional, physical and psychological) and who were unable to reconcile some of the philosophical differences between theory and practice were more likely to discontinue their studies.

While it is clear that there are similarities between the reasons given for discontinuing studies for undergraduates on traditional programmes and professional degrees, the main difference appears to be that nursing and midwifery students tend to be more motivated and committed to their studies. So why do they leave before finishing? The main reason appears to be that nursing and midwifery students are expected to cope with the different learning terrains of the NHS (shift work, dress code, behaviour) and university life (open discussion, study skills, academic rigour). Individuals on professional degrees are more likely to be exposed to situations and events which are both anxiety provoking and physically demanding and therefore more likely to feel stress. Stressful events can leave you with a sense of empowerment and achievement if managed well, or feelings of failure and burnout if not.

Recognising and managing stress in your own life appears to be an important success indicator. Individuals can learn how to manage stress effectively and develop high levels of resilience. Resilience 'is the ability of an individual to positively adjust to adversity' (Jackson et al, 2007: 2). Jackson et al identify that levels of resilience amongst nursing students can be enhanced through fostering nurturing relationships, developing emotional insight/awareness and effective time management to ensure a healthy work-life balance (see the students' accounts of their courses throughout this book).

The following survival tips aim to help you cope with the unexpected, manage change and be accepted into your new group of friends. They will also help you develop informal and formal support networks.

TOP TIPS

- Produce a realistic plan of how you will balance your home and study commitments and manage stress levels (see 'pre-course preparation').

- Don't start your journey if you are already experiencing ill-health, personal or financial problems. Wait until you have resolved these issues.

- Take time to make friends in your group, take regular exercise and maintain a good social/family life away from work.

- If you are living away for the first time don't go home on your days off for the first few weeks as this will increase opportunities for meeting other students, making new friends and enjoying the benefits of university life!

Am I the right kind of person?

In life it is nearly always unhelpful to pigeonhole people into types as this leads to extreme views: good or bad; suitable or unsuitable; hard working or lazy. However, insight into the attributes of successful students can help you recognise your own strengths and weaknesses to maximise your chances of success. Therefore we are going to continue by offering information about *personal attributes* of successful student nurses/midwives for our rucksack.

Current research evidence suggests that successful nursing and midwifery students tend to be:

- aged over 26 years and confident;
- focused but can visualise future possibilities;
- agreeable and conscientious.

Mature and confident

Older and mature individuals appear to cope better with the demands of professional degrees than younger (aged less than 25 years) or immature students. However, while there are some advantages to being an older student, they are more likely to have problems balancing the demands of the course with child care and other domestic responsibilities. So does this mean that if you are 18 and considering a career in nursing or midwifery you shouldn't apply until you are older? The answer is a resounding *no*! Older does not always mean someone is wiser or mature. It is accepted that maturity and age don't necessarily go together, and why everyone over the age of 18 is eligible to apply for a nursing or midwifery course. Now would be a good time to review Martin Spurin's comments earlier in the chapter (see p. 115).

But if you are in the 'younger' student age group then it might help if you gain 'life experience' by undertaking voluntary work in the UK or abroad, or take a gap year. These types of activities will help you gain new perspectives, improve your confidence, demonstrate commitment and help your application to stand out from the crowd. These experiences will also give you something to talk about if you succeed in being shortlisted for a selection day or interview. Students who are confident in their own abilities and who have previously studied in higher education (HE) have been found to be more able to cope with the demands of theory and clinical practice. For obvious reasons students with higher confidence levels and experience of HE were more likely to be in the older age group (Green and Baird, 2009; Yorke and Longden, 2008).

Realising future possibilities

Students who appreciate the benefits of continuation, and who appreciate that the demands of study and financial hardship are time limited are more likely to complete their studies. Juggling the demands placed upon you will require a degree of selfishness (or focus) and an acceptance that you will not be able to completely satisfy everyone while undertaking your education. If you are a perfectionist who is unable to compromise or someone who is selfless then you are less likely to succeed (Deary et al, 2003). Forward planning by asking for help from family and friends will help effectively balance your workload with other commitments. Because of the way degree programmes are designed, students tend to focus their attentions on the semester they are studying or the next assignment deadline. But dividing nursing and midwifery courses in this way can lead to some students getting lost and forgetting why they embarked on the journey in the first place. For these reasons it is important not to forget the reasons why you wanted to embark on your chosen career and to visualise the kind of practitioner you want to be. Keeping a reflective journal can help you think about your own philosophy of care and realise the alternatives to the way care is delivered locally. Reflection can help you visualise the potential possibilities of being a qualified nurse or midwife.

'Getting on and fitting in'

Being a successful student nurse or midwife requires that you 'get on' with patients, clients, doctors and nursing/midwifery mentors. 'Agreeableness' and 'conscientiousness' are terms used by Atkinson et al (1990) to describe individuals who tend to be able to 'get on' with people and who can be depended upon to do the work that they are asked to do. Turning up on time for your shifts and university sessions and being enthusiastic and keen to learn also conveys to others that you are a conscientious student. Many studies have found that new students are often asked by their clinical mentors to perform tasks such as cleaning or tea making (Yearsley, 1999; Jones and Wylie, 2008). These kinds of activities may seem unimportant but willingness to help in this way demonstrates agreeableness and will help you be accepted into the nursing/midwifery team you are assigned to. So if at any time during your first placements you feel at a loss, then offer 'to lend a hand', with bedmaking or other menial tasks. This shows your mentor that you are keen and provides you with important learning opportunities, for example, observing how members of staff interact with patients/clients and gaining insight into the routines of the ward or department.

TOP TIPS

- *Improve your confidence and ability to cope with stressful situations by undertaking voluntary work at home or abroad.*

- *Keep a reflective journal and include your reasons or philosophy of why you want to be a nurse/midwife. Revisit your philosophy at regular intervals to help you think about future possibilities. At the end of each year celebrate what you have achieved.*

- *Ask for help along the way!*

- *Whether you are in university or clinical practice always turn up on time and try not to miss any sessions or shifts.*

- *When you start clinical placements, turn up on time and appear keen and helpful and offer to help with basic tasks.*

Conclusion

Your rucksack is probably feeling a bit heavy by now, but remember that sharing some of this evidence about students who stay on nursing and midwifery programmes will help you develop strategies for becoming a successful student. If you are a mature, hardworking, organised, resilient, agreeable, conscientious individual, then you are very likely to enjoy the challenges and transformational learning that occurs. Many that have started the adventure that you are about to embark on have succeeded and are now helping people like themselves to journey towards professional qualification. As Ernest Hemingway pointed out, 'it's good to have an end to journey towards, but it is the journey that matters in the end'.

Summary

- **It is quite normal to feel anxious about your abilities to be a successful student nurse or midwife. The practical advice and reflections contained within this chapter should help address these concerns, and encourage students to discuss them with each other at all stages of the programme. This serves as an important support mechanism.**

- Nursing and midwifery courses are very demanding programmes, and it is therefore important to consider ways in which you can pre-empt some of those demands and develop strategies that maximise resilience.

- It is vital not to lose sight of your ultimate goal, especially when you have worked so hard to get to this point. By this stage of the book therefore, it is now important to think about *how* you will keep focused on your goal of becoming a registered nurse or registered midwife.

References

Atkinson RL, Atkinson RC, Smith EA and Bem DJ (1990), *Introduction to Psychology* (10th edn). San Diego: Harcourt Brace Jovanovitch.

Bekhradnia B and Bailey N (2008), *Demand for Higher Education to 2029*. Higher Education Policy Institute Report. Available at: http://www.hepi .ac.uk/466-1366/Demand-for-Higher-Education-to-2029.html

Bragg F, Cromwell D, Edozien L, Gurol-Urganci I, Mahmood T, Templeton A and van der Meulen J (2010), Variation in rates of caesarean section among English NHS trusts after accounting for maternal and clinical risk: cross sectional study. *British Medical Journal*, 341: c5065. Available at: http://www.bmj.com/

Deary IJ, Watson R and Hogston R (2003), A longitudinal cohort study of burnout and attrition in nursing students. *The Journal of Advanced Nursing*, 43 (1): 71–81.

Donnison J (1988), *Midwives and Medical Men*. Historical Publications.

Goleman D (1995), *Emotional Intelligence*. New York: Bantam.

Green S and Baird K (2009), An exploratory, comparative study investigating attrition and retention of student midwives. *Midwifery*, 25(1): 79–87.

Jackson D, Firtko A, Edenborough M, et al (2007), Personal resilience for surviving in the face of workplace adversity: a literature review. *The Journal of Advanced Nursing*, 60 (10): 1–9.

Jones C and Wylie L (2008), An exploration of the factors that cause stress to student midwives in the clinical setting. *Midwives online:* October/November. Available at: http://www.rcm.org.uk/midwives/ in-depth-papers

McIntyre H (2011), Midwifery taster course for prospective midwifery students. *British Journal of Midwifery*, 19(1): 57–60.

NMC (2008) The Code: Standards of conduct, performance and ethics for nurses and midwives. Available at: http://www.nmc-uk.org/Nurses-and-midwives/The-code/The-code-in-full/

NMC (2009) Standards for pre-registration midwifery education. Available at: http://www.nmc-uk.org/Educators/Standards-for-education/ Standards-for-pre-registration-midwifery-education/

NMC (2010) Standards for pre-registration nursing education. Available at: http://standards.nmc-uk.org/Pages/Welcome.aspx

Salovey P and Mayer H (1990), Emotional intelligence. *Imagination, Cognition & Personality*, 9: 185–211.

Welton J, Decker M and Adam J (2006), How far do nurses walk? *MedSurg Nursing*. Available at: http://findarticles.com/p/articles/mi_mOFSS/is_4_15/ai_n17214422/

Yearsley C (1999), Pre-registration student midwives: fitting in. *British Journal of Midwifery*, 7 (10): 627–31.

Yorke M and Longden B (2008), *The first year experience of higher education in the UK*. Final Report. London: The Higher Education Academy.

Index

A

B

C

D

E